T0215162

Ronald Jay Werner-Wilson, PhD

Developmental-Systemic Family Therapy with Adolescents

Developmental-Systemic
Family Therapy
with Adolescents

HAWORTH Marriage and the Family
Terry S. Trepper, PhD
Executive Editor

Developmental-Systemic Family Therapy with Adolescents

Ronald Jay Werner-Wilson, PhD

The Haworth Clinical Practice Press
An Imprint of The Haworth Press, Inc.
New York • London • Oxford

Published by

The Haworth Clinical Practice Press, Inc., an imprint of The Haworth Press, Inc., 10 Alice Street, Binghamton, NY 13904-1580

Client identities and circumstances have been changed to protect confidentiality. In some instances, similar cases have been combined to form a composite profile.

Cover design by Jennifer M. Gaska.

Library of Congress Cataloging-in-Publication Data

Werner-Wilson, Ronald Jay.
    Developmental-systemic family therapy with adolescents / Ronald Jay Werner-Wilson.
        p.   cm.
    Includes bibliographical references and index.
    ISBN 0-7890-0118-7 (hard : alk. paper)—ISBN 0-7890-1205-7 (soft : alk. paper)
    1. Adolescent psychotherapy. 2. Group psychotherapy. 3. Family psychotherapy. I. Title.

RJ505.G7 W47 2000
616.89′14′0835—dc21   00-038328

To my wife, Tracey, for all of her love and support

CONTENTS

SECTION III: ADOLESCENT RISK TAKING

SECTION IV: TREATMENT ISSUES

ABOUT THE AUTHOR

Ronald Jay Werner-Wilson, PhD, earned his doctorate from the University of Georgia's Marriage and Therapy program, which is accredited by the American Association for Marriage and Family Therapy (AAMFT). His teaching, research, and clinical experience have all emphasized an interest in adolescence. He began working with adolescents as a youth counselor in 1984 and began clinical work as a family therapist with adolescents in 1990. He has been associated with AAMFT and the National Council on Family Relations since 1990; he is a clinical member and approved supervisor in AAMFT.

Dr. Werner-Wilson is currently the Clinic Director and an Assistant Professor in the AAMFT-accredited Marriage and Family Therapy doctoral program at Iowa State University in the Department of Human Development and Family Studies. He was formerly an Assistant Professor and Clinic Director for the AAMFT-accredited MFT master's program at Colorado State University. He has taught both undergraduate and graduate courses on adolescence and has been conducting research on adolescence since 1988. Dr. Werner-Wilson has two research interests: adolescence and the process of marriage and family therapy.

CONTRIBUTORS

Robert W. Marrs, MS, received his Master of Science degree in Counselor Education from the University of Wisconsin–Whitewater. He is currently a doctoral student in Marriage and Family Therapy at Iowa State University, Ames, Iowa. He is a Clinical Member of the American Association for Marriage and Family Therapy, and a licensed Marital and Family Therapist in the state of Iowa. He has a background in adolescent/family therapy in all levels of care and treatment modalities.

Darren A. Wozny, MA, received his Master of Arts in Marriage and Family Therapy from the University of Louisiana at Monroe. He worked for several years as a family psychologist for Mental Health Services in Canada and maintained an Employee Assistance Program (EAP) private practice. He is currently a doctoral student in the Marriage and Family Therapy program at Iowa State University, Ames, Iowa. He is a member of both the American Association for Marriage and Family Therapy and the National Council on Family Relations. His research interests include: dropouts in couples therapy, supervision practices, and influences of the Internet on couple and family relationships.

Acknowledgments

Developmental-Systemic Family Therapy with Adolescents is the product of interdisciplinary training, multiple sources of professional development, experiences working with adolescents and their families, and supportive personal relationships.

I would like to begin by acknowledging the support and encouragement of professional colleagues. Paula Dressel and Ralph La-Rossa, two early mentors, inspired me to devote my career to the study of families and family relationships. Ralph continues to be a role model of significant import. Sharon Price nurtured me through my doctoral studies and has been an invaluable source of support thereafter. Toni Zimmerman, Ray Yang, Clifton Barber, Maurice MacDonald, Linda Enders, Harvey Joanning, and Jacques Lempers are a few of my many colleagues who have supported this project at various points of development.

Several graduate students have contributed to this project. Megan Murphy invested a significant amount of time locating and obtaining references for this project. Marty Erickson, Miguel Chupina-Orantes, and Jennifer Fitzharris helped identify other important resources. I would also like to thank Jennifer for her editorial contributions.

Robert W. Marrs and Darren A. Wozny agreed to contribute chapters. Their efforts and professionalism are greatly appreciated.

I would like to thank the adolescents and their families who have provided me with the opportunity to learn from them.

Finally, I would like to thank my family for supporting me through the experience of authoring my first book. In the months leading up to completion, the first question my parents or siblings often asked was, "Are you finished with that book *yet?*" At various times, this question provided me with encouragement as well as incentive to complete it. My wife, Tracey, and our children, William and Frances, are sources of personal inspiration. Their invaluable support has sustained me through this effort.

Introduction

Developmental-systemic therapy integrates constructs and research findings from developmental psychology, social psychology, family studies, systemic family therapy, and social constructionism to provide a pragmatic approach to clinical intervention. Understanding ideas from each of these traditions enhances understanding about adolescent development. For example, developmental psychologists have identified various aspects of individual adolescent development—cognitive development, emotional development, identity development, self-esteem—that influence potential presenting problems. These aspects of adolescent development are influenced by parenting style and type of adolescent-parent attachment. Both of these dimensions have been investigated extensively by developmental psychologists. Therapists who understand adolescent development and respond in developmentally appropriate ways to these issues are more likely to experience clinical success.

Various components of adolescent development will be discussed in Section I. Attachment and parenting style will be reviewed in Section II. Throughout this book, aspects of adolescent development that influence common presenting problems are identified and practical interventions that draw from a variety of family therapy traditions are described. Assessment instruments that seem to have clinical utility as well as empirical validation are also identified. Clinical intervention based on this integration of research findings from related disciplines represents a developmental-systemic approach to therapy with adolescents.

Regardless of family therapy theoretical orientation, it is important to understand adolescent development. Clinicians often overlook the special stressors that families of adolescents experience. Adolescents are routinely both gods and ghosts in their family systems and the therapeutic process. Teenagers are often mysterious specters in the therapy room. Jeff, a thirteen-year-old, for example,

1

retreats by moving his chair away from his mother, a single parent; he also avoids eye contact and provides minimal answers to my questions. Adolescents such as Jeff are shadowy figures, particularly if their family has recruited them into the role of identified patient. Many are recruited into this role.

Adolescents may also exert an almost otherworldly control over family systems because they have the unique power to energize a family via potentially fatal disruptive behavior. Adolescents, in contrast to younger children, are more likely to take such risks as driving a car while intoxicated, engaging in unprotected intercourse, and experimenting with alcohol and other substances that impair them. Erin, a fourteen-year-old, sneaks out at night and drives around with her friends. Sometimes they drink or get high, increasing the possibility that they may be injured in a car accident. Chris, a seventeen-year-old, has had several sexual encounters in which he did not use a condom, putting himself at risk for HIV/ AIDS. In addition to engaging in risky behaviors, adolescents are also godlike because they are simultaneously and paradoxically

- wary and sarcastic,
- vulnerable,
- egocentric,
- impressionable,
- stubborn,
- and supremely confident.

Because it may be difficult to work with adolescents and because therapists may not understand adolescent development, some therapists dismiss adolescents from therapy so that they can work on "parenting skills" or "couple issues." As a result, the therapist may not address interaction patterns that contribute to problematic relationships between the parents and an adolescent child.

Developmental themes have not been explicitly addressed in family therapy theory, particularly for this stage of the life span. Some schools of family therapy have suggested that family process is more important than the content of the presenting problem. This obscures, in therapy with adolescents and their families, the impact of particular developmental themes on family process. For example, family relationships influence adolescent self-esteem, which, in turn, influences family interaction; this is consistent with systemic therapies that recognize recursive family relationships. Other family therapy theories, influenced by social constructionism (e.g., narrative therapy, solution-focused therapy), have also ignored developmental themes. Emphasizing postpositivistic themes such as collaboration and a cocreation of reality, these approaches view scholarship on individual human development as prescriptive. Constructionist clinical work is enhanced, however, by an understanding of physical, cognitive, and emotional development. I supervised a case, for example, in which the therapist interacted with a physically mature thirteen-year-old as if he had adult cognitive-processing ability. The therapist became frustrated because the boy did not respond to his constructionist-inspired metaphors and stories. It was obvious that the boy, although physically mature, had not adequately mastered abstract thought; as a result, the therapist had to use more concrete language.

ORGANIZATION OF THE MATERIAL

The book is organized into four major sections. Four categories of adolescent development are discussed in the first section: cognitive development, emotional development, identity development, and self-esteem. The second section reviews three aspects of adolescent interpersonal relationships: attachment, parenting, and peer relationships. The third section examines three types of adolescent risk taking: sexuality, alcohol and substance abuse, and suicide. The final section reviews conceptual information including chapters on use of self and postmodernism. Each chapter features the following:

- Relevance to marriage and family therapy approaches
- Identification of common presenting problems related to the chapter topic
- Case examples
- Treatment issues such as assessment, therapy process dynamics, and interventions

CONCEPTUAL APPROACH

A pragmatic approach to therapy with adolescents is discussed here. Rather than focus on a single theoretical approach to therapy, the utility of tactics from multiple approaches is considered. For example, principles of narrative therapy are incorporated in the chapter on identity development (Chapter 3) and tactics from structural therapy are addressed in the chapter on treatment of alcohol and substance abuse (Chapter 9). These might seem antithetical approaches but each seems appropriate for the respective topic. The use of experiential therapy (Chapters 2, 5, and 8) and solution-focused therapy (emphasized in Chapter 6) are also discussed at length.

ASSESSMENT

Assessment is a common theme in each chapter. Both clinical assessment tactics to use during sessions and self-report measures to provide additional information about a particular aspect of adolescence are identified. Measures that have established psychometric properties that seem to have clinical validity are reviewed. Although these measures are useful tools, they do not replace careful clinical assessment.

SECTION I:
ADOLESCENT DEVELOPMENT

Chapter 1

Cognitive Development

Cognitive development is the first theme from the developmental-systemic model that will be discussed. How does stage of cognitive development affect family therapy? Parents may become frustrated with their children who, entering the formal operations stage, balk at family rules and challenge their parents. Clinicians may become frustrated if they develop vague interventions or use metaphors with an adolescent who, dominated by concrete operations, does not respond to these abstractions. In this chapter, principles of cognitive development in adolescence and clinical implications and assessment of cognitive processing ability are reviewed. Adolescent egocentrism, which is influenced by cognitive development, is also addressed.

INFLUENCE OF COGNITIVE DEVELOPMENT ON THE THERAPY PROCESS

I recently consulted with Sam, a very talented therapist, because he was becoming frustrated with Barry, a thirteen-year-old boy who had been arrested for shoplifting at a local discount store. Sam surmised that Barry was struggling to separate from his family. Sam scheduled individual interviews with Barry so that, as Sam told Barry, they "could brainstorm less problematic strategies to individuate." I was happy that Sam was one of the rare therapists who incorporates aspects of adolescent development into his clinical practice. Sam's hunch about individuation was sensitive to an important developmental construct.

When I met with Sam in his office, the environment seemed pleasant and professional. His diploma hung on a wall over his desk. His license and certificate of clinical membership were tastefully placed on opposite sides of his degree. A computer sat on one corner of Sam's slightly cluttered but organized desk. Sam's two wooden bookcases featured an assortment of family therapy books, which suggested that he was at least familiar with recent developments in the field; most of the books appeared to have been read. A video camera sat on a tripod in one corner of the office. The office reflected Sam's competent demeanor.

As Sam asked me to sit down, his face clouded over. "I'm struggling to connect with Barry. He seems to be acting out in order to distance himself from his parents. His parents are afraid that his behavior will worsen and lead him into more severe trouble. They're fairly authoritarian in their parenting style." I was, therefore, further impressed with Sam's command of adolescent development, but I was concerned about his use of language.

Sam showed me a video clip in which he attempted to "re-author Barry's story." Sam said to Barry, "I wonder if you shoplift because you want independence? Do you take things because you want to show that you can take care of yourself?"

Barry shrugged. "I don't know. Maybe. I hadn't thought about it."

Encouraged by Barry's tentative agreement, Sam attempted to externalize the problem: "What would you call this part of yourself that seeks to separate from your parents, this part that seeks to separate in ways that are problematic?"

"I'd call it shoplifting," Barry replied. Sam seemed irritated and the session stalled.

The session may have stalled for two developmental reasons. First, the intervention—reflective questions—were not developmentally appropriate for a twelve-year-old. Second, Sam's language may have been too abstract. Scholars influenced by social constructionism suggest that language fundamentally influences therapy. A narrative approach, for example, suggests that problem-saturated stories contribute to and maintain difficulties. In this case, Sam appropriately identified important developmental themes, but he neglected to take into account Barry's stage of cognitive development. It is quite likely that the intervention would have been a success with a slightly older adolescent who was capable of abstract thought, but, because Barry seemed to be in the concrete operations stage, the session stalled.

I observed a case at our clinic in which one of our graduate students made the opposite error. She was working with a seventeen-year-old adolescent girl and her family. The girl had recently been in trouble for breaking a series of rules. The therapist surmised that family rules needed greater clarity and initiated a session in which consequences were jointly negotiated by the parents and the girl. The therapist hoped that this activity would "give the daughter more ownership of the rules," but it didn't seem to help. In this case, the adolescent, who is older than the boy from the previous example, didn't want "arbitrary rules." Although she had helped construct consequences, she didn't approve of the "family rules which they [her parents] made." In this case, it was more helpful to negotiate more than consequences: the young woman, entering the formal operations stage, wanted to create rules as well.

PRINCIPLES OF COGNITIVE DEVELOPMENT

According to noted Swiss psychologist Jean Piaget, cognitions are mental processes that help us acquire knowledge. Cognitions organize our thoughts and experiences because they influence our perceptions, which, in turn, affect the meanings we attach to those perceptions. Piaget proposed a *readiness* model to explain learning behavior: children and adolescents are unable to learn something unless they have achieved a particular stage of development. There are two learning procedures: *tutorial* and *self-discovery*. Dominant educational and parenting models are based on a tutorial approach: learning is directed by adults who establish formal or informal learning goals and methods to achieve them. Learning that occurs spontaneously or because of personal initiative is known as self-discovery. It is more effective than a tutorial approach (Brainerd, 1978).

Assimilation and Accommodation

Observers either assimilate experiences into their existing view of the world or, as a result of information that challenges it, their view of the world is changed, which is referred to as accommodation. Cinical conversations such as narrative or solution-focused questioning and interventions such as reframing are often designed to promote accommodation. Therapists seek, particularly when working from social constructionist orientations, to help people see their lives or their problems in new ways. Adolescents might, for example, resist family rules because, in part, they believe that the rules are unfair and arbitrary; also, these adolescents might believe that their parents are malicious in their attempts to "control" their behavior. Therapy could focus on suggesting to the adolescents that the rules reflect the parents' concern and love rather than maliciousness. The adolescents might also be offered the chance to negotiate "fair" rules. Both interventions focus on helping the adolescents change their perception of the situation.

Attempts to foster new perceptions are thwarted by assimilation. The adolescent described in the preceding example may not accept the therapist's reframe and may be unwilling to negotiate new rules. Why? Why is assimilation such a strong, and frustrating, part of adolescence? Potential answers are available by assessing stages of cognitive development.

Stages of Cognitive Development

Piaget and his colleague Barbel Inhelder, in their book *The Growth of Logical Thinking from Childhood to Adolescence* (Inhelder and Piaget, 1958), suggested four stages of cognitive development—sensorimotor, preoperational, concrete, formal—but adolescents are likely to operate within the latter two, concrete or formal, so concentration is focused on these two stages. Adolescents who emphasize concrete operations are dominated by rules, while those who rely on formal operations are able to consider abstract concepts.

The concrete operations stage begins around age seven or eight and is considered part of the transition to the formal operations stage, which is the final stage of operational intelligence. Charles Brainerd wrote one of the more comprehensive reviews of Piaget's work on cognitive development, titled *Piaget's Theory of Intelligence* (1978). According to Brainerd, during the concrete operations stage

- mental operations are only possible when they are applied to information from direct experience;
- relationships between objects are seen as constant, so there is a tendency to understand the concept of *conservation* between

objects (e.g., if two different-shaped glasses are filled with the same amount of water from one source, the child will be able to recognize that the same amount is in each glass);
• rules are developed to explain principles of conservation (e.g., the original amount of water poured into a container is more important than the shape of the container); and
• there is a tendency to place objects and experiences in some kind of order (e.g., from small to large, young to old) or category (e.g., color, sex).

Stages of cognitive development are often described as distinct from one another, but according to Brainerd (1978), although the formal operations stage begins between the ages of eleven and twelve, it is not solidified until about the age of fifteen. This suggests that younger adolescents may use concrete operations in some situations but formal operations in others. The formal operations stage is associated with the ability to

• consider possibilities,
• test hypotheses,
• plan for the future,
• be introspective, and
• consider and expand beliefs.

General Treatment Implications Associated with Stage of Cognitive Development

In general, it may be helpful to "normalize" problems associated with cognitive development to parents. Family conflict may be reduced if clinicians discuss parental expectations about adolescents in each cognitive stage and to "normalize" (a solution-focused intervention), aspects of the specific cognitive stage. It may be useful to coach parents to use language that is compatible with stage of development.

Some therapy models are better suited than others to working with adolescents in each stage of cognitive development. For example, abstract interventions (e.g., externalizing a problem) may help adolescents in formal operations but frustrate adolescents in concrete operations. It is important to assess an adolescent client's stage of cognitive development. Pay attention to language. Does the adolescent use metaphors and abstract concepts (formal operations) or rely on precise words (concrete operations)? Do rules provide the adolescent with a sense of continuity (concrete operations) or frustration (formal operations)?

Concrete Operations: Common Presenting Problems and Treatment Implications

Adolescents in concrete operations may begin to struggle at school on assignments that require abstract thought. For example, a single mother named Frances sought therapy for her thirteen-year-old son, Jeff, who had recently been suspended from school for truancy. He had been skipping his English literature class. Frances indicated that she was frustrated with Jeff because "He doesn't apply himself. He only seems to do well in classes that are interesting to him. He's got to learn that you have to apply yourself in all areas. I can't tell my boss that I don't want to work on a project because it's boring!"

Jeff's truancy could be related to a number of causes, such as peer influence (Chapter 7), self-esteem (Chapter 4), individuation (see Chapters 3, 5, and 6), or cognitive ability to complete assignments. These other dimensions will be addressed in later chapters. I assessed each of these dimensions to varying degrees and decided to focus on cognitive themes.

"Is that right, Jeff?" I asked. "Are you skipping English because it's boring?"

"Yeah," he answered.

I was not surprised that Jeff did not elaborate on his own, so I asked, "What bores you about the class?"

"It's stupid. The stories are stupid and the homework is stupid. Who cares about the French Revolution?"

"Which classes are interesting? Do you do well in them?" I asked.

He thought for a moment and replied. "Science is pretty cool. I like the labs. I'm pretty good in algebra too."

"What are your grades in those classes?" I wondered.

"That's the frustrating part," Frances exclaimed. "He's doing great in those classes. It's almost like he has dual personalities."

This information, an exception to Jeff's problem behavior, suggested that skipping class might be specific to the course, rather than Jeff's ability. I surmised that Jeff was probably dominated by concrete operations and wondered if the assignments in history and English frustrated him because they required more abstract thinking.

"Why are the assignments stupid?" I asked.

Jeff replied sarcastically, "'Describe the symbolism associated with Valjean's theft of a loaf of bread. How does the theft reflect the oppression of the masses?' What the hell kind of a question is that? Why doesn't she just ask questions that make sense?"

It would have been a plausible approach to focus on the influence of Jeff's friends who did encourage him to skip class. It was also tempting to concentrate on the theme of individuation. It seemed, however, that Jeff's decision to skip class might be related to the type of assignments that required a level of abstract thinking that frustrated Jeff. Since Jeff performed well in math, we worked to turn the assignments into logic problems: "Why is bread important? Why did Valjean steal the bread? Was his arrest and punishment appropriate? Do you think that others were arrested for similar kinds of crimes? Since his crime was similar to others, does it represent a pattern of injustice?"

In addition to academic difficulties, family conflict may be influenced by aspects of concrete operations. Older siblings who are in concrete operations may seek to enforce family rules during the absence of parents, which could lead to sibling conflict. Fourteen-year-old Steve, for example, told his eleven-year-old brother Mitch to get his feet off the table. "Who are you, my mother?" Mitch asked sarcastically. The argument escalated and the boys broke a lamp while wrestling. Ann, their mother, hearing the disturbance, entered the room and yelled at them to "stop fighting." Steve tried to explain, "Mitch had his feet on the table and wouldn't take them off." Ann replied, "Next time, come tell me. It's not your job to discipline your brother." Frustrated, Steve yelled at his mother.

Why was Steve frustrated? On other occasions, he had gotten in trouble for not telling his mother when Mitch did something wrong, and he had also gotten in trouble for "tattling" on his brother. Trying to make sense of his mother's responses, which were different depending on mood, timing, and situation, was frustrating for Steve because he seemed to want a clear rule structure. This is consistent with concrete operations.

Family rules may be another source of conflict for adolescents in concrete operations if rules are not clearly identified. Exasperated parents often ask their adolescent, "Why did you do that?" and their level of exasperation may increase when the child replies, "I don't know." It's quite likely that adolescents *are* unaware of their motivation; they may also be confused about specific implications of abstract rules. I often work with parents and adolescents in this stage to develop specific rules and, when appropriate, consequences. It is impossible to establish a rule for everything, so parents may need to be coached to help adolescents identify specific implications of general rules. I encourage parents to be very specific about expectations or rules.

In addition to sibling conflict and misunderstandings about rules, parents of adolescents in concrete operations may experience frustration because children complain that parents are unfair. A fifteen-year-old, for example, may become angry if a younger sibling is allowed to engage in an activity (e.g., wearing makeup) at an earlier age. For their part, younger children in concrete operations may complain that an older sibling's increased responsibilities and privileges are unfair.

For adolescents in the concrete operational stage, make linkages between interventions and goals explicit. Solution-focused, problem-focused, and other goal-directed, behaviorally oriented models seem useful. Structural interventions are also helpful. In the case study presented at the beginning of this chapter, the therapist struggled with Barry because his language was not developmentally appropriate. Clinicians should use language that is as precise as possible. If there is any question about comprehension, seek clarification. Many therapists mistakenly seek clarification by asking an adolescent client, "Do you understand?" This is a mistake because the adolescent may be embarrassed to admit that he or she did not understand. Say, instead, "I'm not sure if I'm being clear enough. Would you tell me how you interpret what we've been talking about?"

Formal Operations: Common Presenting Problems and Treatment Implications

Adolescents in the formal operations stage may resist rules that they consider unfair. Reggie is an example. His mother contacted me because Reggie, who was seventeen years old and had never before been in trouble, was suspended from school for stealing. Reggie, who was legally blind (he had limited vision), was an avid sports fan who served as a coach's assistant for the high school football team. Reggie took a pass key from the coach's desk without asking so that he could fulfill his responsibilities more efficiently. "I got tired of asking the coach for a key so I could get a piece of equipment. When I saw the key laying on the desk, I took it. He got another one, so it was no big deal." Reggie used the key for one year before he was caught using it to take a shortcut in the main school building. "I got tired of always walking around this section, which was supposed to be for teachers only. I used my key to get through." Reggie, who seem to be solidly in formal operations, rebelled against what he considered to be arbitrary rules. To his way of thinking, students should be allowed to have school keys in order to do their jobs, so the theft, and subsequent use of a short cut, were justified.

Interventions with adolescents in formal operations should encourage self-reflection and collaboration between therapist and adolescent client. Family interventions should include opportunities for the adolescent to negotiate rules. Family conflict may increase when adolescents enter formal operations and begin to challenge parental authority. As I worked with Reggie's family, for example, I also discovered that Reggie and his stepfather regularly argued about rules. Again, Reggie found the rules to be unfair: "It's his way or the highway. Why is he always right?" We worked together to establish a rule-making structure in which Reggie was given the opportunity to negotiate rules and consequences.

ADOLESCENT EGOCENTRISM

The terms "ego" and "egocentrism" are misused in casual conversation to describe a person who is thought by an observer to be too proud, too selfish, or too arrogant. For example, one teenager may comment to another, "He's just so full of himself. Just because he's student body president. What an ego!" I have also had conversations with clinicians who have misused the term in this way.

Developmental psychologists use the term differently: *egocentrism* is formally defined as "a lack of differentiation in some area of subject-object interaction," and it takes a unique form in each stage of cognitive development (Elkind, 1967, p. 38). This definition suggests that children and adolescents master some aspect of their world in each stage of development. For example, children in the sensorimotor stage (younger than two years) learn to distinguish between self and objects such as their bottle or their parents. According to David Elkind (1967) egocentrism in adolescence requires distinguishing between one's own thoughts and others' thoughts and is demonstrated in two unique ways known as *imaginary audience* and *personal fable*.

Imaginary Audience

Adolescents who enter formal operations are able to consider abstractions and possibilities; initially, this ability to form abstractions and possibilities may lead them to believe that others have the ability to know what they are thinking, so the adolescent becomes increasingly self-conscious. This heightened self-consciousness has been called imaginary audience. Imaginary audience refers to an adolescent's belief that others are preoccupied with his or her behavior. Young children sing, play, and experiment with limited self-consciousness. In middle school, this changes: adolescents are less inclined to try new behaviors and are often reluctant to perform publicly because they are afraid they might do something embarrassing.

This contrast was particularly striking in the T family. Mindy, a thirteen-year-old, was initially an unwilling therapy participant at our campus clinic because we videotape our sessions and all of our rooms feature one-way mirrors. She sat with her back to the mirror and I noticed that she kept glancing up at the camera that was pointed toward her. It was likely that her self-consciousness exacerbated her nervousness about them so we talked about the use of the camera. I told her that she would have the right to meet anyone who observed (all clients have this right but I emphasized the point to Mindy) and offered to let her spend some time in the observation booth experimenting with the equipment. She gradually became more engaged in therapy as time progressed and she became more comfortable with the mirrors and cameras. Her three sisters (ages six to eight), on the other hand, were active and engaged from the very beginning of therapy. I suspected that this difference was the product of heightened self-consciousness due to Mindy's concern about an imaginary audience.

The power of the imaginary audience is influenced by school and family structures because teachers and parents—who are part of a *real* audience—monitor adolescent behavior. This monitoring intensifies self-consciousness: adolescents who perceive that their parents are supportive are less self-conscious, but if adolescents perceive rejection from their parents, self-consciousness increases (Riley, Adams, and Nielsen, 1984). The family has an interesting influence on girls' imaginary audience: self-consciousness is reduced if girls perceive an affectionate relationship with their parents (Adams and Jones, 1982). The influence of parental supervision on imaginary audience is demonstrated in the case of Catherine. Catherine described her mother, Mable, as intrusive. "She [Mom] reads my diary, notes from my friends, and tries to listen in on the phone when I'm talking to my friends. I don't have any privacy. I get tired of her spying on me and getting me in trouble." Mable would also drive around their small town looking for Catherine's car to see if Catherine "was where she said she'd be."

Mable was a concerned parent who was worried about her daughter because of material she read and conversations she overheard. Her concern influenced her to vigilantly monitor Catherine, which, in turn, seemed to cause intense conflict between the two. Ben, the father, responded to the conflict by punishing Catherine. Mable's monitoring and Ben's punishment increased Catherine's self-consciousness. Catherine responded by becoming increasingly belligerent and hostile. This relationship cycle exemplified the axiom that "the solution can become the problem." This case is discussed further in Chapter 4 concerning self-esteem and suicide.

Imaginary Audience: Treatment Implications

As with cognitive development, it might be helpful to normalize to parents the increased self-consciousness associated with imaginary audience. It might also be helpful to identify relationship cycles that unintentionally increase the self-consciousness of an adolescent in the family. In cases where this may occur, possible cycle-breakers could include asking both parents and adolescents to develop new responses.

Don and Michelle demonstrated a problematic relationship cycle that was exacerbated by Michelle's self-consciousness. Don, Michelle's stepfather, would look over her shoulder while she was doing a math assignment. She would impatiently tell him to "stop hovering" because "it made her nervous." He would respond by pointing out an error. She would become frustrated and, according to Don, "stomp off to her room." We developed several cycle-breakers that provided both with an opportunity to end the cycle. Don agreed to ask Michelle if she wanted help rather than provide unsolicited advice. Michelle indicated that if she wanted help, she would not wait for Don to give her an answer. Also, she suggested that "it would probably help if I ask him to help me solve the problem rather than ask him, 'Is this right?' "

Intense self-consciousness can be debilitating because adolescents may not try new activities which, in turn, may negatively influence their self-esteem, which may further heighten self-consciousness. Encouraging adolescents to look for opportunities to take limited risks may be a way to break this particular cycle. Michelle, from the preceding example, risked asking Don, who could be quite caustic, for help. By coaching him to be less critical, we hoped her requests might encourage her to take risks in other parts of her life.

In therapy, clinicians should also recognize that self-consciousness might negatively influence participation of adolescents, especially during the early stage of treatment. We should remember Mindy, the thirteen-year-old who was sensitive to the cameras and one-way mirrors, and attempt to make our adolescent clients less self-conscious about therapy process.

Personal Fable

Personal fable, the second manifestation of adolescent egocentrism, refers to feelings of uniqueness that are often associated with feelings of invulnerability and enhanced risktaking. This phenomenon may influence two sets of problems. First, parents may inadvertently damage their relationship with adolescent children because they fail to recognize the level of seriousness their child attaches to a problem. For example, a parent who tells a child that he or she is overreacting or "going through a phase" may embarrass the child, who may then be reluctant to trust the parent with future disclosures.

After Samantha's parents died in an automobile accident when she was twelve, she moved south to live with Stella, her maternal aunt, and George, Stella's husband. Stella and George were Samantha's only living relatives. The couple had limited experience with children and reported that they struggled to cultivate a relationship with Samantha. George told me, "Samantha is driving me crazy. She's so moody."

"How is she moody?" I wondered. "Can you give me a specific example of this moody behavior?"

"Okay." George thought for a moment and continued. "Okay. Last week she came home from school crying because her boyfriend had broken up with her. Now, I don't usually get into this kind of thing but Stella wasn't home so I thought I'd try to give her some comfort. When she told me that Jim, or whatever his name is, had broken up with her, I told her that she'd get over it because it seemed like a silly schoolgirl crush. Then she yelled, 'God, I hate you. Why are you such a jerk?' and stomped off to her room."

From George's perspective, the incident was trivial. It typified an infatuation of limited consequence. His attempt to comfort Samantha, by telling her that she would "get over it," might have made Samantha angry because she perceived George's comfort as invalidating.

Family conflict, the second type of problem associated with this phenomenon, may increase because adolescents may resist family rules. This resistance to rules is different from the resistance discussed earlier in the chapter. That resistance focused on adolescents' questioning of rules they considered to be unfair or arbitrary. Resistance associated with personal fable is different: adolescents may underestimate threats to their personal safety.

This aspect of personal fable was exemplified in the case of Dan, a fifteen-year-old boy, who had been arrested for breaking into an automobile. It was not his first delinquent act; he had been previously arrested for shoplifting. The family had consulted with a family therapist after the shoplifting incident but Lisa, Dan's mother, reported, "Nothing really changed. Dan doesn't seem to understand the consequences of his behavior." When I consulted with Dan, he did, indeed, seem unimpressed with the seriousness of his situation. "It's no big deal," he said. His mother yelled back, "What do you mean it's no big deal? You've got a criminal record now!" Dan shrugged. "So?" he asked rhetorically. My task was to help Dan see that his behavior and the consequences of his actions were relevant in order to address feelings of invulnerability associated with personal fable.

Personal Fable: Treatment Implications

Working with adolescents requires constant vigilance to the context and interpretation of the problem. For example, normalizing some concerns might empower an adolescent to take a limited risk. This would positively address self-consciousness. One should be cautious, though, because the adolescent might experience the intervention as a sign that "you don't understand" the significance of the issue. As a result, I tend to use tentative language with adolescents. I generally say something like, "I'm feeling pulled in a couple of directions. On one hand, this seems to be a significant problem for you and I want to hear more about its significance. On the other hand, I know that a lot of people struggle with this, and I don't want you to feel like you're weird or different because you're having these feelings." Hopefully, this kind of statement addresses self-consciousness by noting that others struggle with similar issues while simultaneously recognizing its significance in order to address feelings of uniqueness.

SUMMARY

Stage of cognitive development influences family relationships and might be associated with a variety of presenting problems. Clinical observation of language and behavior provides clues to stage of development. Interventions and treatment process should be adjusted to accommodate adolescents who are in either concrete or formal operations. Furthermore, therapists should be sensitive to two manifestations of adolescent egocentrism: imaginary audience (increased self-consciousness) and personal fable (feelings of uniqueness).

Chapter 2

Emotional Development

Emotional development is the second theme from the developmental-systemic model that will be discussed. Emotional development is another aspect of adolescence that has a significant impact on family dynamics, presenting problem, and therapy process. The following is reviewed:

- Aspects of emotion
- Developmental issues
- Emotion in families
- Emotion in family therapy

In their book *Emotion in Psychotherapy*, Leslie Greenberg and Jeremy Safran (1987) conclude that emotion is adaptive and fused with cognition and behavior: "Emotion is a fundamental aspect of human experience. The problems that bring people to psychotherapy rarely, if ever, stem from problems in cognition or behavior, independent of emotion" (p. 6). Researchers Robert and Anita Plutchik (1990) have studied the adaptive functions of emotions and make the following assertions:

- Emotions are adaptive because they provide important information.
- Emotions have a genetic basis.
- Emotions are subjectively experienced, and interpretation and response are influenced by cultural norms and attitudes about emotional experience and response.
- Emotions are influenced by feedback and contribute to a complex chain of events.

These assertions are clinically relevant for understanding emotional development in adolescents. Although young children learn rules of emotional expression (e.g., "boys don't cry"), adolescents must incorporate a much more sophisticated set of rules that are related to cultural norms. Additionally, self-consciousness (see Chapter 1) may increase the intensity of emotions during adolescence. Parents take for granted rules of emotional expression, so they may be insensitive to emotional development in adolescence. It may be helpful to remind parents of the adaptive and subjective nature of emotions.

THREE ASPECTS OF EMOTION

Researchers have concluded that emotions are experienced physiologically; this physiological stimulus is interpreted and responded to subjectively (Hatfield and Rapson, 1990; Saarni and Crowley, 1990). In this section, three aspects of emotion are reviewed: *biological, cognitive,* and *behavioral.*

Biological Aspects of Emotion

Researchers have convincingly demonstrated that there is a physiological basis for emotions. For example, chemicals that occur naturally in the brain produce emotions (Hatfield and Rapson, 1990). Emotions also produce facial reactions that, although outwardly masked, can be detected with electromyogram (EMG) readings. Recognizing that there is a physiological aspect of emotion is clinically relevant. Although one is unlikely to conduct a chemical analysis or an EMG reading of one's clients, this line of research suggests that careful attention should be paid to emotions:

- Some models of therapy completely neglect emotions, but, because they are a fundamental part of the human experience, clinical skills that respond sensitively to emotions should be cultivated.
- Parents, who may be more skilled at managing their own emotions, may not recognize the significance of adolescents' emotional responses.
- Adolescents may require assistance in sorting out and responding to conflicting feelings.

Cognitive Aspects of Emotion

Although there is a physiological basis for emotions, we experience them subjectively for two reasons: (1) rules associated with emotions are learned, so they are influenced by culture and family norms, and (2) emotions are idiosyncratic experiences. Intense emotional experiences seem to interfere with our ability to cognitively process emotions: "[W]hen people are caught up in an intensely emotional situation, 'chemical spill-over' is likely to occur—that is, peoples' feelings get all mixed up. Everything gets intensified. . . . They know that they are feeling intensely but it is difficult to disentangle their complicated interlocking feelings" (Hatfield and Rapson, 1990, p. 17). In the earlier clinical example, Samantha's request for support rather than protection seems to exemplify her need to understand her feelings.

Behavioral Aspects of Emotion

Some responses to emotion may be innate. For example, the "fight or flight" response to distress, and comfort seeking (e.g., infant sucking behavior), seem to be a part of our genetic makeup. These are behavioral responses to emotion. Rules associated with emotional expression influence many behavioral responses, so they are learned. Clinically, it seems important to help families negotiate behavioral responses because of differing expectations associated with them.

DEVELOPMENTAL ISSUES

Themes associated with emotional regulation that seem to be influenced by development are reviewed next. Carolyn Saarni and Michael Crowley (1990) make two propositions about emotional regulation:

1. Emotional regulation is influenced by rules for emotional expression that become more complex during adolescence.
2. Emotional regulation influences coping with stress.

In addition to reviewing these two aspects of emotional regulation, aspects of cognitive development that are likely to influence emotional development are briefly discussed.

Rules for Expressing Emotions

Saarni and Crowley (1990) suggest that emotional development becomes more sophisticated with age; adolescents are more likely than younger children to mask their feelings because their social world is more complicated. In many cases, adolescents are expected to act emotionally indifferent. This rule seems to be strongest when adolescents are in the company of peers and it comes at a cost: adolescents, especially boys, are expected to suppress genuine feelings.

Working with families, it might help to remember that emotions provide important information to all members of the family and that feedback in families influences emotional experience. Families often have communication rules. Plutchik and Plutchik (1990) suggest that families also have rules about emotional expression. It may be helpful, then, to inquire about these rules.

Emotional rules seemed to contribute to family conflict for Samantha, the young woman discussed in Chapter 1 who moved in with her maternal aunt, Stella, and Stella's husband, George, following the automobile accident that killed her parents. George reported that he was frustrated with Samantha's "moodiness." When he attempted to comfort Samantha after her boyfriend ended their relationship by telling her that she would "get over it," Samantha became angry. In the earlier chapter, I suggested that Samantha became upset because she thought that George trivialized the significance of her emotional pain. I also wondered if George and Stella might have adopted a family prohibition about sadness as a way to protect Samantha.

To investigate this possibility, I asked a fairly open-ended question about emotional rules. "What happens when someone in your family is sad?"

"We try to cheer them up," Stella replied. George nodded in agreement. Samantha remained silent. This seems to be a fairly common emotional rule that is inspired by a desire to inoculate family members against negative feelings. In doing so, though, this rule may interfere with emotional expression. From a Mental Research Institute (MRI) perspective, this could be an example of an attempted solution becoming a problem.

I probed with another question. "Samantha, how do you feel about their attempts to cheer you up? Is this something you want?"

"No," she exclaimed loudly. "Why do I always have to be happy? If I feel bad, can't I just feel bad?"

I turned to Stella and George. "I suspect that you're trying to 'protect' Samantha. Is that right?"

This time George answered. "Of course we're trying to protect her. She's been through so damn much. Isn't that what you do for someone you love? Don't you try to protect them from getting hurt?"

"Samantha, do you want to be protected? Or would you rather have their support and understanding when you're sad?"

"I want the support and understanding. Because they're always trying to cheer me up, I feel like it's not okay to be sad or frustrated. I have to be some kind of happy robot."

George looked puzzled so I asked Samantha to elaborate. "Can you explain the difference? I think that George and Stella want to help."

"Could you just listen to me without trying to solve my problem?"

This clinical example demonstrates the significance of emotional expression to adolescents, as well as family rules that may interfere with it. Later in this chapter, several approaches to help families become more comfortable dealing with emotions are reviewed.

Emotions and Stress

Saarni and Crowley (1990) also propose that emotional regulation influences ability to cope with stress. This seems particularly important for adolescents who experience stress as a normal part of their development. Stress is associated with identity development, interpersonal demands (e.g., friendship, dating, peer pressure), academic responsibilities, extracurricular obligations, and family relationship patterns (e.g., divorce, remarriage). Some adolescents may respond to stressful situations by ignoring their emotional response, so they might not seek support from others.

Recall from Chapter 1 the case of Jeff, who began to skip his English literature class. Jeff may have struggled in the class because, dominated by concrete operations, he found the material too abstract, so we worked to turn abstract questions into solvable problems. In this case, the problem was exacerbated because Jeff seemed reluctant to seek help. He reported that he was upset about the course, but he did not seek help from the teacher, his mother, or the school counselor. Because this seems fairly common, therapists might want to help students who regulate emotions by ignoring them to become more aware of their emotions and to seek help from others when they are feeling overwhelmed.

At the other end of the continuum, some adolescents may over-react to stress by turning normal stressors into catastrophes. Parents, who may become frustrated by this heightened emotional sensitivity, may respond dismissively to the child. This parental response may exacerbate the problem because the child, feeling invalidated, may become even more emotional.

In each case, emotional regulation influences an adolescent's response to stress. Careful attention should be paid to the interrelationship between emotional regulation and response to stress so that appropriate responses can be made. Parental responsiveness and family rules about emotional regulation should also be investigated.

Influence of Cognitive Development
on Emotional Development

Recall Hatfield and Rapson's (1990) warning that intense emotional experiences create a "chemical spill-over" that is difficult to interpret. Heightened self-consciousness associated with egocentrism may exacerbate this intensity. Coping with intense emotions and stress as well as interpreting emotional rules is likely to be influenced by stage of cognitive development.

For example, adolescents in concrete operations who rely on a rule-based cognitive structure may experience frustration trying to figure out emotional rules that are often inconsistent. Clinically, one would want to help these adolescents develop a menu of responses to emotionally challenging situations. On the other hand, adolescents in formal operations who rely on abstract thinking and meta-rules may experience intense emotions in a more personal manner.

EMOTION IN FAMILIES

Carolyn Saarni and Michael Crowley (1990), in their review of emotional regulation, suggest that families fundamentally influence emotional development: "Our implicit and explicit relationships with others are a powerful tool in influencing what we express" (p. 62). For example, Saarni and Crowley note that research on child abuse suggests that children who experience abuse are more likely than those who have not experienced abuse to demonstrate avoidance and denial of negative emotional states. Hatfield and Rapson (1990) suggest that family members have the following influence on emotions: (1) ability to express emotions with clarity, (2) intensity of response to emotions, and (3) ability to interpret the emotional expression of other people.

Support in Families

Families are a primary source of support. This support includes an emotional component that has been discussed by Thomas Wills (1990). He discusses two positive aspects of family support and identifies five mechanisms that promote support.

Positive Aspects of Support

First, Wills suggests that family support may reduce negative feelings which, in turn, influences positive self-feelings (e.g., enhanced self-esteem) and creates a climate of mutual support in the family. Second, Wills proposes that family support may promote health-protective behavior. People who experience support engage in regular conversation with others, so they are more likely to identify physical problems and seek medical attention.

Mechanisms of Support

First, research suggests that family members support one another by confiding in one another. Second, problem-solving activities contribute to an atmosphere of support. Third, families help adolescents learn specific coping skills. Fourth, parental support networks provide support for children. Finally, family members serve as an anchor against negative messages from peers and the media.

Given the importance of family support, it should be assessed regularly. Clinically, each of the five mechanisms of support identified by Wills (1990) can be evaluated. There are also self-report measures that assess dimensions of family support. The McMaster Family Assessment Device, which measures multiple dimensions of family functioning, will be discussed in Chapter 6. Four of the subscales could be used to assess the following mechanisms of support: communication, affective responsiveness, and affective involvement.

Intimacy in Families

Intimacy is typically a topic of concern in conjoint couple therapy, but it is also relevant in family therapy with adolescents because of adolescents' continuing need to feel connected to their parents. This connection is an intimate one. Elaine Hatfield and Richard Rapson (1990) describe three characteristics of intimacy: *cognitive, emotional,* and *behavioral:*

1. *Cognitive Characteristics:* willingness to reveal oneself to another when there is reciprocal self-disclosure within an ongoing relationship. This may be particularly important during adolescence as the relationship between parents and children shifts from unilateral to mutual in nature.
2. *Emotional Characteristics:* willingness to reveal, the cognitive dimension, is influenced by perception of trust and intensity of feelings in the intimate relationship. Due to self-consciousness (discussed in Chapter 1), adolescents are quite sensitive to emotional experiences that adults may trivialize; this may damage trust between adolescents and parents. Establishing trust is a particularly significant goal in earlier stages of therapy; it should be ensured that all participants in therapy share a sense of trust.
3. *Behavioral Characteristics:* affectionate gestures contribute to intimacy in families and are easily observed. Attention to seating arrangements and other structural characteristics provides important information about this characteristic of intimacy. Does the adolescent sit closer to one parent than another or does he or she withdraw from all relationship contact? How do family members use eye contact and other nonverbal gestures to communicate emotions such as support or empathy, rejection or anger?

Improving Intimacy in Families

Hatfield and Rapson (1990) recommend four strategies to improve intimacy in family relationships:

1. Encourage self-acceptance
2. Encourage acceptance of differences in others
3. Encourage communication of ideas and feelings
4. Promote nondefensive listening skills

Encourage self-acceptance. I have noticed that parents and adolescents who have difficulty in this area have trouble accepting differences in others, which, in turn, is associated with increased family conflict. Thus, self-acceptance of all family members should be assessed. (This could be done with the Rosenberg Self-Esteem Inventory, which will be discussed in Chapter 4.)

Encourage acceptance of differences in other family members. Parents who are poorly differentiated (Rob Marrs discusses differentiation in Chapter 11) may interpret adolescent individuation as a sign of rejection. Perception of parental support influences adolescents in many ways, so it is important to spend time assessing and enhancing acceptance of others.

Encourage communication of ideas and feelings. Adolescents regularly tell researchers and clinicians that they would like to have conversations with their parents that are more mutual in style. They report that their parents are more likely to lecture them than to talk to them. It is important to assess the manner in which parents and adolescents communicate and to promote a climate in the family that is receptive to reciprocal exchanges. Parenting style (see Chapter 6) significantly influences communication patterns.

Promote nondefensive listening skills. Nondefensive listening skills can be cultivated in several ways. Many psychoeducational approaches seem to work with some clients. In other cases, awareness of reactivity may help members listen. Hatfield and Rapson note that, at times, one person will say something or communicate a feeling that others in the family will not like. In these cases, the speaker should try to communicate her or his own emotional response in a way that does not attack or invalidate others. This is, of course, influenced by self-acceptance and acceptance of others.

Parents often ask adolescent children variations of "why" questions. Robert and Anita Plutchik (Plutchik and Plutchik, 1990) suggest these questions are likely to increase defensiveness and impair intimacy in relationships. Additionally, people have difficulty answering "why" questions because of limited self-awareness. This may lead to many other problems.

EMOTION IN FAMILY THERAPY

Greenberg and Safran (1987) suggest that emotions should receive significant attention in therapy because many problems are related to blocking or avoiding emotional experiences. Assessment and discussion of emotional content can help clients face problems that have been avoided. Greenberg and Safran also propose that processing emotional experience produces a shift in the nature of emotional experience, which may, in turn, lead to client change. According to their review of the literature, research seems to support these two propositions.

Doherty and Colangelo (1984) suggest that some models of family therapy are better suited to address affect, such as Bowenian family systems therapy, symbolic experiential family therapy, and emotionally focused therapy. Major features that seem salient for use in family therapy with adolescents will be discussed, but many other excellent volumes are available on each approach.

Bowenian Family Systems Therapy

Family therapist Murray Bowen concluded, after twenty years of studying families and practicing family therapy, that most human activity is governed by emotions and postulated that emotional fusion can impair intellectual functioning (Bowen, 1978). Edwin Friedman, in his review of Bowenian family therapy, elaborated on the importance of *family emotional systems,* which are defined as a group of people who have developed emotional interdependencies (Friedman, 1991). Emotional systems include the following:

- The members' thoughts, feelings, emotions, fantasies, associations, and past connections (individual as well as group connections)

- The members' physical makeup, genetic heritage, and current metabolic state
- Each individual sibling position and parents' sibling positions
- The emotional history of the system itself

A Bowenian approach to family therapy emphasizes differentiation. Therapists are encouraged to cultivate differentiation from their own families as they simultaneously coach their clients to differentiate as well. Differentiation is a concept that seems to be misunderstood. Often, differentiation is described as a process of seeking independence or individuation from one's family of origin. This does not seem to be Bowen's intent, because he often emphasized emotional interdependence. He suggested that individuals need to experience both togetherness and individuality (Bowen, 1978). Friedman (1991) elaborates: "self-differentiation is the process of getting in touch with intergenerational processes, to know them, to experience them, and to be emotionally affected by them" (p. 148). This is not a state of emotional detachment for therapist or client.

Symbolic Experiential Family Therapy

Symbolic experiential family therapy emphasizes confronting emotions as a central part of therapy. Carl Whitaker and David Keith (1991) describe the role of therapists in symbolic experiential family therapy:

- Therapist serves as a coach or surrogate grandparent to the family.
- Therapist is active in therapy process. They suggest that the therapist should infiltrate the family and expose anxiety-laden territory.
- Therapist encourages the family to set goals and to be active.
- Self-disclosure of therapist is part of the process. The therapist should seek to be congruent with her or his clients.

The final role, self-disclosure of the therapist, is a critical element in this approach. Robert Marrs' excellent discussion of the use of self (Chapter 11) is a valuable resource for working with adolescents. Before discussing a more systematic approach to integrating emotions in therapy, aspects of what Keith and Whitaker (1987) refer to as a "personal" self in therapy will be discussed briefly. They suggest that a personal self is

- critical of social norms and willing to raise questions;
- creative, spontaneous, unpredictable;
- willing to risk ridicule by acting silly;
- willing to use unconscious associations;
- potentially dangerous;
- inconsistent; and
- engaged in a constant growth process.

Emotionally Focused Therapy

An emotionally focused approach to therapy systematically addresses emotion in therapy. This approach is based on several postulates (Greenberg and Safran, 1987). First, emotion, cognition, and behavior are interdependent. Second, cognitive-affective experiences are adaptive. Third, the adaptive function of emotion is primarily interpersonal. Fourth, emotional experience involves synthesizing information that is both internal and external. Fifth, emotion is a form of tacit knowing. Finally, emotional experience is linked to personal identity.

Greenberg and Johnson (1988) developed a framework for integrating emotions in systemic therapy with couples. Because the steps in their approach seem to have merit for addressing affect in families as well, the steps that they recommend and specific techniques to address emotions in therapy are reviewed.

Step one: identify conflict issues. In this step, the therapist is encouraged to frame problems in terms of emotional pain, deprivation of emotional bonds, and insecure attachment. *Step two:* identify negative interactional cycles. *Step three:* access unacknowledged feelings. *Step four:* redefine the problem(s) in terms of underlying feelings. *Step five:* promote identification with disowned needs and aspects of self. *Step six:* promote acceptance. *Step seven:* identify personal needs. *Step eight:* identify new patterns of interaction.

Discussion of specific interventions to address emotions is rare in marriage and family therapy. Greenberg and Safran (1987) provide a systematic approach to dealing with emotions in therapy; following is a brief review of their seven specific strategies:

1. *Attending:* encourage the client to pay attention to underlying feelings and needs
2. *Refocusing:* redirect the client back to internal, subjective feelings about his or her experiences
3. *Present-centeredness:* help the client to focus on the present emotional experience rather than past experiences
4. *Expression analysis:* point out nonverbal aspects of expression as a source of information about emotional response
5. *Intensifying:* increase vividness of experience by promoting emotional or physical arousal
6. *Symbolizing:* use of metaphors to help create a more vivid understanding of emotions
7. *Establishing intents:* after clarifying affect, ask clients what they would like to do

SUMMARY

Emotional development is intertwined with cognitive development. Both aspects influence family relationships, presenting problems in therapy and therapy process. Assessment should include attention to emotional expression in families such as family rules about emotional expression, emotional regulation, and intimacy in families. Techniques from experiential and humanistic approaches to family therapy with adolescents help families cultivate emotional intimacy. Additional chapters on attachment (Chapter 5) and the parent-adolescent relationship (Chapter 6) will address aspects of family interaction and family therapy that promote emotional connection in families.

Chapter 3

Identity Development

Identity development is the third theme from the developmental-systemic model that will be discussed. Why should a family therapist be concerned about adolescent identity development? Family conflict may escalate if parents and adolescents have different short- and long-term goals and aspirations. Humans require both connectedness and separation, a paradox that is clearly evident during adolescence. Melissa, a fifteen-year-old, reports that her parents are often intrusive and embarrassing. "I hate the way they dress and Dad can be so corny when my friends are around. He tells stupid jokes and teases us." Still, Melissa also acknowledges that when she is feeling really lonely or afraid she seeks her mother.

Identity and identity development have received significant attention from developmental psychologists, social psychologists, and sociologists, but this work is often neglected in the family therapy literature. The work of developmental psychologists may have been ignored because the two themes that have dominated family therapy—systems theory and social constructionism—seem incompatible with some of the *language* used to describe identity development. Erik Erikson's psychosocial perspective, for example, is based on a stage approach to identity development that might *appear* to be incompatible with tenets of systemic or social-constructionist approaches to therapy.

Although family therapists have neglected the formal construct referred to as identity development, the importance of identity has not been lost on family therapists who have substituted constructs such as "dominant story," "interactional rules," "multiple realities," and others to describe dimensions of identity. If a pragmatic approach to helping adolescents is adopted, it seems important to explore aspects of identity development that may enhance our systemic and social-constructionist approaches to therapy.

It seems ironic that family therapists have neglected the writing of developmental psychologists because the latter have incorporated ideas that are consistent with family therapy ideas. In the *Handbook of Child Psychology,* the preeminent reference on child development, Harold Grotevant (1998) suggests that a narrative approach to identity development facilitates understanding of "how the different domains of identity are related to one another, and particularly how domains of identity that are assigned are related to those that are more freely chosen" (p. 1123). Grotevant continues by noting identification of reconstructed stories, a narrative tactic, is "a key to understanding current functioning" (p. 1123).

The term "identity," like many psychological constructs that take on a life of their own in casual conversation, is often misused and misunderstood. What is identity? What is the function of it? What seems to influence adolescent identity development? Addressing these questions is the first step toward understanding an important aspect of adolescence.

WHAT IS IDENTITY?

James E. Marcia (1980) describes identity as "an existential position . . . an inner organization of needs, abilities, and self-perceptions" (p. 159). He also proposes that identity is a socially constructed, dynamic structure: "an internal, self-constructed, dynamic organization of drives, abilities, beliefs, and individual history. . . . The identity structure is *dynamic, not static*" (p. 159, emphasis added). Sociologist Charles Horton Cooley (1902/1956) suggested that people use a *looking glass self,* the perception of how one is perceived by others, for self-evaluation. Clearly, these two definitions are compatible with a social-constructionist perspective.

Gerald R. Adams suggests that identity has two dimensions: *personal* and *social.* Adams (1976) writes, "Personal identity can be seen as a fusion or summation of membership roles, past and present identifications, and personal character, all of which are united by a cognitive network structure and are summarized by the person into *self-definitions*" (p. 151).

Adams' definition is consistent with systemic and social-constructionist principles. For example, "membership roles" and "past and present identifications" suggest that family interactions influence an individual. Likewise, Adams notes that identity is based on "self-definition," which is compatible with social constructionism. Social identity, the second dimension of identity, refers to statuses and roles that an individual assumes in a social context. This idea, too, is consistent with social constructionism.

IDENTITY CRISES

Both Marcia and Adams are influenced by the psychosocial perspective of adolescence developed by Erik E. Erikson. Erikson suggested that identity development is a lifelong process that is based on the resolution of eight major crises or dilemmas. According to Erikson (1968), adolescents must resolve two dilemmas:

- Industry versus inferiority
- Identity versus role confusion

Industry versus Inferiority

Children and preadolescents between the ages of seven and eleven confront the first adolescent dilemma: industry versus inferiority. This refers to awareness of a sense of achievement and familiarity with social expectations. "How do you know if a girl likes you?" Jordan, a ten-year-old, once asked me. I consulted with Jordan and his family because his parents were concerned that Jordan "wasn't fitting in." I worked with the family for a few sessions to help both the parents and Jordan adapt to this normal dilemma of identity development.

Parents usually respond when their adolescent children experience academic difficulties. This attention may help their children respond positively to feelings of inferiority that are likely to accompany the problem. Parents may not understand nor respond when children experience feelings of inferiority because of academic *success*. Troy, another early adolescent, had difficulty at school. Although he received high grades, he struggled to fit in because his classmates teased him. Although he had mastery in a cognitive domain, Troy struggled to obtain mastery in the social domain.

Troy is like many bright students. His academic achievement seemed to block his social growth. Troy asked for concrete strategies to help him make more friends (peer relationships will be discussed at length in Chapter 7). I asked him to describe a day at school. Troy, perhaps because he wanted to demonstrate achievement in some area of his life, taunted his classmates about grades. He described a fairly common pattern. A teacher would distribute a test and he would ask others, "What grade did you get?" They would tell him and he would show them his grade, which was usually much higher. He would then ask them to tell him what problem or question they had missed and would act surprised and say, "How could you miss such an easy question?"

Bright adolescents such as Troy are often teased because their peers feel threatened by them. This suggests, however, that the interaction is one-sided and that all bright students are doomed to social isolation. Troy's description of a typical day suggested that he participated in the process. By taunting his classmates about their grades, Troy seemed to contribute to their feelings of inferiority which, in turn, resulted in Troy being treated badly.

Students such as Troy can be taught social skills. I tend to frame them as problems to solve so that adolescents can use their cognitive mastery to solve social problems. For example, I asked Troy if his classmates might feel insulted by his incredulous question, "How could you miss such an easy question?" or if he bragged about his grades.

"I guess so."

"Let's try to solve this problem," I suggested. Using a solution-focused intervention, I imbedded a presumptive question in the following homework assignment: "What will you do differently the next time your teacher returns an assignment so that you don't insult others? What will you do to make a friend instead?"

Troy was enthusiastic when he arrived for our next session. "I figured out the answer to your problem," he said. "Instead of bragging about my grade, I asked the guy next to me if he'd like any help figuring out a homework answer. A couple of days later he asked me if I wanted to play soccer with him."

Identity versus Role Confusion

Middle and late adolescents are more likely to be preoccupied with integrating various identifications from childhood. This crisis is described as identity versus role confusion and includes development of self-confidence, a sense of purpose, and a cohesive self-perception. To successfully complete the task of identity development, Erikson suggests that adolescents should have cultivated trust, autonomy, initiative, and industry from earlier stages. Identity development may contribute to various problems between adolescents and their parents and, Gerald Adams (1976) suggests, is related to egocentrism (as we discussed in Chapter 1, this refers to heightened self-consciousness and enhanced risk taking) as well as level of cognitive development.

According to Erikson, resolution of this crisis is reflected in attempts to answer the question, "Who am I?" and he warns that adolescents who are unable to answer this question are in danger of adopting a "negative identity" such as "delinquent," "troublemaker," and "druggie." Adolescents who are socially isolated at school or serve as family scapegoats are at particular risk for developing a negative identity. In April 1999, two high school teenagers shot and killed twelve classmates and a teacher at a suburban high school in Littleton, Colorado. As they opened fire on their classmates, it was reported they targeted "jocks" as well as minorities. One of the teenagers reportedly had a brother who was considered a successful high school athlete before he graduated, while the other attacker was described as being socially isolated. So, for different reasons, each boy adopted the persona of a group known as the "Trenchcoat Mafia," which provided a sense of identity.

Leslie, a fifteen-year-old girl, is another example of someone who adopted a negative identity. I consulted with Leslie and her family after Leslie had completed a ninety-day inpatient program for substance abuse. Leslie described herself as a "misfit" in high school and her parents told me that they were surprised by Leslie's drinking problem. Leslie's mother said, "We had no idea that she was going to parties to get drunk. She had been spending so much time alone in her room that, frankly, we were relieved that she was starting to become more socially active." Substance abuse is further addressed in Chapter 9, so I will focus only on the identity crisis aspect of Leslie's drinking problem in this chapter.

I was concerned that Leslie used the term "misfit" to describe herself: "How are you a misfit?"

She responded, "I don't fit into any of the groups at school. I'm not a jock; I'm not in the band; and I'm not smart enough to be a brain. . . . Isn't that weird, geeks have more friends than me." Leslie seemed to demonstrate role confusion: she identified different groups at school but was unable to see herself as fitting into any of them. Attending parties and becoming intoxicated became her identity: "I was a primo party girl," she said with a mixture of pride and shame.

IDENTITY STATUS

Identity provides a sense of personal control (e.g., internal versus external locus of control), personal meaning, and personal identification. James Marcia (1980) developed a typology to describe identity status. Each stage is influenced by family relationships and features unique psychosocial characteristics, demonstrating the recursive link between individual development and interpersonal relationships. Each stage is distinguished by two factors: (1) the presence or absence of a decision-making period (referred to as a time of crisis) and (2) the extent of commitment to occupation and ideological goals (Marcia, 1980). Marcia identified four statuses:

1. Identity achievement
2. Moratorium
3. Foreclosure
4. Identity diffusion

The following discussion about identity status is based on James Marcia (1980) and Susan Harter's (1990) summary of research on identity statuses.

Identity Achievement

This identity status represents the ideal form of identity resolution and refers to people who have experienced a period of decision making and have independently chosen occupational and ideological goals. The following characteristics are associated with this status: self-reflection, future orientation, productiveness, and independence. Individuals in this status are less likely to conform to peer pressure than individuals in other statuses, are socially adept, demonstrate a deep commitment to relationships, and are warm and compassionate.

Although this may be an "ideal form" and the attributes associated with it are positive, it is possible that this status could provide conflict between adolescents and parents if an adolescent's commitment to an occupation and ideology differ significantly from the family's. For example, Joan wanted to major in English literature but her parents wanted her to study business. Her parents convinced her to take business classes before changing majors. Joan successfully completed classes in marketing and accounting but she reported that she still wanted to major in English literature. I consulted with Joan and her parents because her father threatened to withdraw financial support. In another case, conflict erupted in a family because the values associated with the ideological commitment of a seventeen-year-old boy were in conflict with the father. The boy and the father engaged in heated disagreements about politics.

Moratorium

This identity status refers to individuals in the midst of a struggle involving either career or ideological goals who are experiencing an identity crisis. Due to the ambiguity associated with this decision-making process, individuals in this status are likely to experience a high degree of anxiety and demonstrate a high degree of rebelliousness. Despite experiencing anxiety, these individuals usually have a stable sense of self-esteem and are likely to use socially mature influence or persuasion.

The anxiety and rebelliousness associated with this status may be related to family conflict. For example, families may have difficulty dealing with a "moody" adolescent, or parents may become concerned when their child begins to break family rules. It may help to normalize (a solution-focused tactic) this anxiety. Parents who are uncomfortable with emotions may have difficulty accepting anxiety as normal.

Parental response to rebelliousness associated with this process of decision making may be problematic. Some parents may interpret rebelliousness as a challenge to parental authority while others may interpret it as a rejection. Parents who adopt an authoritarian parenting style (parenting styles are discussed in detail in Chapter 6) and respond harshly to normal acts may contribute to the problem.

Although rebelliousness is a normal part of this identity status, it is important for clinicians to distinguish between behavior that is associated with this decision-making process and problem behavior associated with other causes. Assessment of identity status, developmental stage, parenting style, and other developmental factors will help distinguish between problem behavior and boundary testing.

Foreclosure

This identity status refers to people who have chosen occupational and ideological goals prescribed by their parents or other authority figures. These adolescents are quiet and industrious but immature. On the surface adolescents in this stage seem placid because they are typically cautious and dependent on others. These adolescents and young adults may begin to struggle in classes that require critical thinking because, due to their limited experience making decisions, they often lack problem-solving skills. Finally, foreclosed adolescents are often moralistic and rigid, so they may have difficulty cultivating and maintaining intimate relationships. These characteristics may also make foreclosed adolescents vulnerable to recruitment by cults or extremist organizations.

Identity Diffusion

This identity status refers to adolescents who have not experienced a decision-making period and have not chosen occupational and ideological goals. The following characteristics are associated with this identity status: feelings of inferiority, alienation, and ambivalence; poor self-concept; high impulsivity; immaturity; uncooperativeness; manipulativeness; susceptiblity to peer pressure; socially withdrawn. These characteristics are part of normal development during early adolescence but may create difficulties in later adolescence.

Although these characteristics are normal for early adolescents, they may contribute to family conflict and academic difficulty. For example, early adolescents who are uncooperative, immature, and impulsive may have difficulty completing tasks assigned in school or may "forget" household chores. It may help families that include younger adolescents if we normalize these behaviors. Behavioral interventions (e.g., development of a chore list), structuring tasks (e.g., reframing, boundary making), and experiential exercises (e.g., enactment, role playing) may help change behavior. Solution-focused interventions (e.g., search for exceptions, the formula first session task) are also developmentally appropriate interventions for adolescents exhibiting these particular characteristics.

Adolescents who are socially withdrawn, feel inferior to their peers, and have a poor self-concept may have difficulty making friends. If these adolescents internalize their social relationships as rejection they may respond aggressively at home by picking fights with siblings or becoming argumentative with parents. In these cases it may be helpful to attend to both family interactions and peer relationships. The first step might be to address family conflict but after the conflict in the home seems to be managed, it might be helpful to normalize the adolescent's response to peer rejection and help the adolescent cultivate social skills.

Older adolescents who remain in a diffused identity status experience a different set of difficulties. For example, an older adolescent who continues to be impulsive, uncooperative, and immature may have difficulty maintaining a job or experiencing success at school. Insight-oriented interventions may be more appropriate than behavioral ones for older adolescents who have not experienced a decision-making period and who lack vocational and ideological commitments. Clinicians could help facilitate exploration of career options and values.

Influence of Parenting on Identity Status

As previously discussed, identity includes a social dimension, so examination of social influences on identity status seems appropriate at this point. Earlier in this chapter, I suggested that humans require both connectedness and separateness. Based on her extensive review of research on identity, Susan Harter (1990) concludes that "identity formation is facilitated by individuated family relationships characterized by both separateness, which gives the adolescent permission to develop his or her point of view, and connectedness, which provides a secure base from which to explore outside the family" (p. 383). This idea is consistent with research on attachment relationships, which will be discussed in Chapter 5.

If we adopt a systemic perspective, it is logical that parenting style influences identity development. Thus, if an adolescent seems to have problems associated with an identity status it seems reasonable to assess parenting style. Although parenting styles are examined at length in Chapter 6, a brief review of parenting influences is presented here.

Democratic Parenting

Democratic parenting is associated with the identity achievement status: the parent-adolescent relationship includes regular praise and interactions with parents as well as negotiation between parents and children. Successful resolution of the moratorium status is associated with a democratic style of parenting: parents who encourage autonomy and self-expression help their adolescent children move from moratorium to achieved status.

Authoritarian Parenting

Authoritarian parenting seems to promote identity diffusion: parents of adolescents in the foreclosed status are often intrusive, indulgent, and possessive of their children. Interventions with parents of foreclosed adolescents may focus on parenting strategies that are more nurturing and promote decision making by the adolescent.

Permissive Parenting

Permissive parenting also impairs the process of identity development: parents of adolescents in the diffused status are often rejecting, detached, and provide limited guidance to their children. Interventions with parents of diffused adolescents may encourage greater parental involvement. A clinical example may illustrate this point.

David, a thirteen-year-old boy, once told me that he had "cool parents" because they did not enforce a curfew: "There are a lot of things that I don't like about my parents, but at least they don't nag me about being home on time. They don't care what time I come home." This boy reported that he had few friends and used negative comparisons to others when he described himself. Remembering that he was socially isolated, I asked him to repeat his description of his parents: "My parents are pretty cool about curfew. They don't care what time I come home."

Something about the way he said the second sentence caught my attention so I commented: "On one hand, your parents are 'cool about curfew' but you also said that they 'don't care.' Your face looked sad when you said that your parents don't care." David began to cry.

Although his parents were "cool," he experienced their attitude about curfew as indifference because, as he told me a little later, "at least my friends who have parents who nag them about curfew know that their parents give a shit about them!" Therapy featured a variety of systemic (e.g., establishing household rules such as a curfew) and insight-oriented (e.g., asking David to explore career interests) interventions to help facilitate both independence and connectedness in the family.

Assessment of Identity Status

Accurate assessment of identity status is an important clinical concern because the characteristics of impulsiveness, uncooperativeness, and immaturity associated with diffused identity status could be misdiagnosed as symptoms of attention deficit disorder. Marcia (1966) developed a formal procedure to identify identity status, but the coding procedures require trained personnel.

Adams and colleagues developed the Ego Identity Scale, another measure of identity status. Clients complete the measure developed by Adams so it is more efficient to administer. Research suggests that the Ego Identity Scale measures each of the identity statuses as well as Marcia's observational measure. To obtain a copy of the scale and scoring information, contact Gerald R. Adams.[1]

DEVELOPMENTAL ASPECTS OF IDENTITY

Self-evaluation and *integration of multiple roles* seem to be influenced by developmental stage. We will review the influence of age on these two aspects of identity development.

Self-Evaluation

Adolescents engage in self-evaluation to provide judgments that affect identity. These judgments seem to be influenced by developmental stage. William Damon, Director of the Stanford Center on Adolescence, and his colleague Daniel Hart of Rutgers University suggest that self-judgments in early adolescence rely on social comparison but self-evaluation in later adolescence is based on personal beliefs and internalized standards (Damon and Hart, 1988). This suggests that attempts to help adolescents resolve identity conflicts should be sensitive to the developmental stage of the adolescent client. We could help younger adolescents choose appropriate sources for comparison (e.g., encourage a seventh grader to compare his or her soccer skills to those of other seventh graders rather than juniors or seniors). On the other hand, identity problems with older adolescents would be best addressed by examining internalized standards that may be inappropriate.

Integration of Multiple Identities

Integration of multiple identities is an important part of adolescent development: social context influences behavior of adolescents, so, in a sense, an adolescent has multiple selves. In her review of the literature on this process, developmental psychologist Susan Harter (1990) concluded that adolescents need to integrate multiple aspects of self into a coherent and unified identity. This aspect of identity development seems to be influenced by developmental stage.

Younger adolescents develop the cognitive skill to recognize inconsistencies in self (e.g., that they are nice to some people and mean to others) but they lack the cognitive skill to make comparisons about these differences. Middle adolescents, on the other hand, seem significantly bothered by these inconsistencies because they develop the cognitive capability to develop a higher order system of abstraction that includes the ability to evaluate these inconsistencies. Older adolescents continue to develop more sophisticated cognitive skills so they are able to *differentiate* between these aspects of self and, as a result, experience less distress about them.

This suggests that problems associated with integration are likely to be different for adolescents based on their developmental stage, therefore interventions should be sensitive to these differences. In particular, this is more likely to be a problem for middle adolescents, so therapy might focus on developing more sophisticated levels of abstraction to enable the client to accept aspects of self that seem contradictory. The following narrative tactics could facilitate identity integration: questioning (especially meaning and preference questions), re-membering, re-authoring, and externalizing aspects of self (Madigan, 1997; White, 1995, 1997; White and Epston, 1990).

Ideal versus Real Self or Actual Self

In addition to developing an integrated sense of self that is associated with multiple roles and contexts, adolescents seem to make distinctions based on discrepancies between an *ideal self,* a *real self* (sometimes referred to as "actual" self), and a *false self.* Ideal self refers to a perception of what one wants to be or beliefs about what one should be. Real self refers to an individual's perception of his or her actual attributes. False self refers to acting in ways that do not reflect the real self. Children begin to make distinctions between parts of self during middle childhood. Research conducted by Susan Harter and colleagues suggests that distinctions between an ideal and actual self are meaningful to adolescents (Harter et al., 1996).

Adolescents describe the real self as

- "the real me inside"
- "my true feelings"
- "what I really think and feel"
- "behaving the way *I* want to behave and not how someone else wants me to be" (Harter et al., 1996)

Adolescents describe the false self as

- "being phony"
- "putting on an act"
- "expressing things you don't really believe or feel"
- "changing yourself to be something that someone *else* wants you to be" (Harter et al., 1996)

Adolescents seem to interpret discrepancies in three ways: (1) devalue real self or experience alienation from real self; (2) engage in false self behavior to obtain acceptance of parents or peers; and (3) engage in multiple roles as part of experimentation. According to Harter and her colleagues, these three interpretations are influenced by perceived support, and they predict false self behavior. Adolescents from the first two groups, those who experience a sense of alienation or routinely engage in false self behavior to please others, report more problems than adolescents who define discrepancies as experimentation. These adolescents are less cheerful, more hopeless, more likely to engage in false self behavior, report lower self-worth, demonstrate higher self-blame, and think more often about suicide (Harter et al., 1996). Their sense of alienation seems to be influenced by family and peer relationships: "It appears that adolescents who report the constellation of conditional support, a low level of support, and hopelessness about support are driven to engage in false behavior in an attempt to try to please parents and peers" (Harter et al., 1996, p. 371).

Because this set of identity difficulties is influenced by perception of support, it seems plausible that intervention should be multidimensional. We previously identified narrative tactics that might help adolescents integrate multiple aspects of self. Those same tactics might help adolescents identify alienated aspects of self in order to resist problem-saturated narratives. It seems, though, that some effort needs to be made to address social support. Structural interventions such as reframing, restructuring, and unbalancing relationships that contribute to a sense of conditional support in the family may reduce an adolescent's perception that he or she needs to please others. In some cases, it may be helpful to assess the influence of family coalitions on perceived support and intervene as appropriate.

Although alienation from self is, as we previously noted, associated with a variety of problems, discrepancy between real and ideal self can have a positive function: it may serve as a source of motivation. People may "actually produce discrepancies by creating challenging standards that mobilize them toward a goal; goal attainment then reduces the discrepancy, leading the person to set even higher standards" (Harter, 1998, p. 575). This suggests that discrepancies between real and ideal self could be used to encourage change in adolescents and their families. For example, solution-focused interventions (e.g., normalizing a discrepancy, identifiying behaviors that are consistent with real self) could be used to identify behaviors that are consistent with real self and to encourage clients to continue to act on their goals.

SUMMARY

Identity development is a process that includes personal and social dimensions that both influence and are influenced by family relationships. Like cognitive development, identity development may be associated with a variety of presenting problems. Assessment of new adolescent clients should include some attention to identity crisis, identity status, developmental aspects of identity, and family factors associated with identity development. Interventions and treatment process should be sensitive to age and level of cognitive development.

Chapter 4

Self-Esteem

Self-esteem, the fourth theme from the developmental-systemic model, significantly influences adolescents. The following factors associated with self-esteem are reviewed:

- Developmental influences
- Domains of importance
- Presenting problems
- Assessment
- Locus of control

In his book *The Antecedents of Self-Esteem,* Stanley Coopersmith (1967) suggests that individuals with high self-esteem have confidence in their decisions, are more aware of their opinions, and are more willing to defend their ideas. In contrast, people with low self-esteem are more self-critical and expect that others, in turn, will be critical of them. Coopersmith concludes: "By dwelling on their ineptitude and insufficiencies, those low in self-esteem are exacerbating their point of greatest sensibility and, at the same time, reducing their opportunity for obtaining success" (p. 69). This suggests that self-esteem provides feedback that reinforces self-perception.

Further research suggests that self-esteem has a significant impact on people. In a series of research studies on adolescents, Susan Harter demonstrated that low self-esteem is associated with depression, which, in turn, is associated with suicidal ideation (Harter, 1993; Harter and Marold, 1993). In addition to influencing depression, self-esteem is a powerful force in the life of adolescents:

• Adolescents with higher self-esteem are less likely to have mental health problems.
• Adolescents with higher self-esteem demonstrate more mature intimacy skills.
• Adolescents with higher self-esteem show more initiative.
• Adolescents with higher self-esteem are more accepting of differences in others.

WHAT IS SELF-ESTEEM?

Research suggests that self-esteem significantly affects the life of adolescents, but what is it? Self-esteem, according to L. Edward Wells and Gerald Marwell (1976) in their monograph of the same title, is "a deceptively slippery concept about which there is a good deal of confusion and disagreement" (p. 5). They note that the concept is widely used but suggest that there is confusion about its meaning for the following reasons:

• A variety of terms (e.g., self-acceptance, self-worth, to name only two) have been used to describe it.
• Researchers and clinicians emphasize different aspects of it, which creates conceptual confusion. The problem is made worse because professionals often use vague language to describe it.
• Casual usage in conversation interferes with precise usage. Because "of the deceptive impression that everyone already knows what self-esteem is, there is a tendency to treat the concept as an independent 'given' " (p. 9).

PRIMARY ASPECTS OF SELF-ESTEEM

Given this state of confusion, self-esteem is defined and aspects of it are discussed here to provide greater clarity. Wells and Marwell (1976), after exhaustively reviewing the literature, suggested that there are two primary aspects of self-esteem: (1) evaluation and (2) emotional experience. Each dimension has clinical implications.

Wells and Marwell refer to the evaluation aspect of self-esteem as *self-acceptance*. Adolescents, influenced by increasing self-consciousness (see Chapter 1), are often preoccupied with self-evaluation. They seem to rate almost every activity. Brandon, for example, told me that his life "sucked." "Why does your life suck?" I would ask and Brandon would recount his struggles in a variety of areas. It seemed that Brandon might feel better about himself if he could identify positive aspects of his life, so I decided to utilize this process of ongoing self-evaluation to try to identify them.

Since Brandon seemed well aware of his behavior and was engaged in evaluating it, I was tempted to use the solution-focused formula first session task (see de Shazer and Molnar, 1984, for a detailed description of this intervention). I decided against that particular intervention, though, because I wanted to avoid trivializing Brandon's experience (see Chapter 1 for a discussion of the influence of egocentrism on therapy process). Instead, I decided to adopt another solution-focused tactic: I asked Brandon to describe aspects of his life and waited for him to describe positive events and experiences. I would ask follow-up questions to these naturally occurring exceptions to his perception that "life sucked."

Wells and Marwell describe *self-love* as the emotional aspect of self-esteem. This aspect is influenced by evaluation that occurs as part of the self-acceptance dimension. For example, Brandon once told me, "I could really do a lot better in school. A lot better. I feel like such a failure." This example included an evaluation dimension ("I could do better") and an emotional dimension ("I feel like a failure") of self-esteem.

Since these two dimensions are interdependent, it is quite likely that addressing one aspect of self-esteem will influence the other. When addressing a particular aspect, it may be helpful to develop a treatment approach that is sensitive to level of cognitive development. For example, the evaluation dimension reflects an instrumental type of activity that may be best addressed from theoretical approaches such as cognitive-behavioral, solution-focused, problem-focused, or some combination of the three. This approach would be more appropriate for younger adolescents who continue to rely on concrete operational thought. The self-love dimension, on the other hand, reflects more of an expressive/affective aspect of experience. As a result, it might be useful to use therapeutic approaches that promote awareness or insight when addressing self-love.

DEVELOPMENTAL ASPECTS OF SELF-ESTEEM

Self-esteem declines during early adolescence but improves and stabilizes during later adolescence. This decline is associated with predictable aspects of adolescent development. For example, change in physical development and transition to middle school are sources of stress and anxiety which, in turn, seem to lower self-esteem during early adolescence. Given the difficulties associated with lower self-esteem that we previously discussed, it may be helpful to normalize this change for adolescents and their families. In addition, the impact of self-esteem on adolescents seems to be influenced by age, stage of cognitive development, and egocentrism. Harter and Marold (1993) summarize this process:

- As an adolescent becomes more self-aware, self-conscious, and introspective, the importance of self-esteem increases.
- As it increases in importance, an adolescent becomes more aware that self-esteem is influenced by social support. Parent support influences self-esteem of younger adolescents who have a need to remain connected to their parents.
- The impact of peer support on self-esteem increases "dramatically" for older adolescents.

These developmental differences suggest that one should respond differently to adolescents according to their age group. For younger adolescents, assess family support, and for older adolescents, assess peer support.

DOMAINS OF SELF-ESTEEM

Self-esteem, in earlier research and common usage, has been defined as a global sense of self-worth. Recent investigators have suggested that self-esteem is influenced by context and interpretation of the context by an individual. Although experiencing success is often associated with high self-esteem, research suggests that the value of success is subjective. Higher self-esteem is associated with both valuing success in a particular area and then experiencing success in that area. Adolescents seem to experience lower self-esteem when they struggle in areas that are important to them.

FACTORS ASSOCIATED WITH SELF-ESTEEM

Physical Appearance

According to a series of studies, perception of physical attractiveness seems to be the strongest predictor of self-esteem in adolescents (Harter, 1993; Harter and Marold, 1993). Susan Harter, who has conducted a series of research studies on self-esteem in adolescence, has concluded that perceived support from parents and friends seems to influence the importance of physical attractiveness. Harter's conclusion seems significant because if physical attractiveness alone predicted self-esteem, intervention would focus on either

• changing physical appearance of the adolescent; or
• changing the adolescent's attitude about physical appearance.

Harter's research, which suggests that it would be inappropriate to encourage adolescents to change their physical appearance in order to improve self-esteem, is consistent with the work of clinical psychologist Mary Pipher. In her best-selling book, *Reviving Ophelia,* Pipher suggests girls who experience eating disorders are preoccupied with physical appearance and resort to dangerous eating habits to change their physical appearance. "Girls compare their own bodies to our cultural ideals and find them wanting. . . . In all the years I've been a therapist, I've yet to meet one girl who likes her body" (Pipher, 1994, p. 184). In my own clinical experience, I have seen a similar phenomenon with adolescent boys who abuse steroids or laxatives (a common practice in the sport of wrestling).

Although it may be helpful to encourage adolescents to change their attitudes about physical appearance, Harter's research suggests that we should address adolescent clients' perception of support from parents and peers. According to Harter, physical appearance does not directly influence self-esteem; instead it is mediated by perception of parent support. Figures 4.1 and 4.2 demonstrate the difference.

Figure 4.2 suggests that adolescents' perception of support is the key element between physical appearance and self-esteem, so intervention should focus on improving perception of support. This finding is consistent with a family systems approach to clinical intervention. The level of parent and peer support needs to be assessed to

FIGURE 4.1. Direct Effect of Physical Appearance

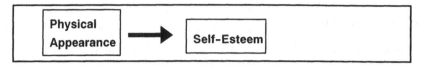

FIGURE 4.2. Physical Appearance Mediated by Perceived Support

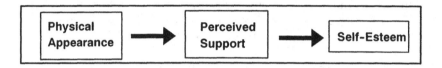

intervene and enhance support, and to see if the adolescent's experience of support increases. For various reasons, changes in tangible support may not be interpreted as a change by the adolescent.

Family Influences

It has been mentioned that parents influence the self-esteem of adolescents (e.g., adolescent perception of support from their parents mediates the influence of physical appearance on self-esteem), but specific aspects of the parent-adolescent relationship associated with self-esteem have not yet been discussed. Morris Rosenberg, who has conducted extensive research on self-esteem in adolescents, has concluded that the type of interest parents show in their adolescent children seems to influence self-esteem (see Rosenberg, 1963, 1979). For example, Rosenberg demonstrated that adolescents were more likely to have lower self-esteem if parents did not show interest in the adolescents' friends, grades in school, or in talking to them during meals. Subsequent research has demonstrated other family influences: family cohesion promotes positive self-esteem (Cheung and Lau, 1985) and excessive parental pressure to succeed has a negative impact on self-esteem (Eskilson et al., 1986).

In his book on self-esteem, Stanley Coopersmith (1967) studied family relationships of high self-esteem children and identified three conditions in their homes. First, parents clearly communicate acceptance. Second, parents set clear boundaries and hold high expectations for their children. Third, parents demonstrate respect for uniqueness and individuality. In addition to these three conditions, Coopersmith identified four factors that contribute to self-esteem, which describe aspects of the parent-adolescent relationship:

- Experience receiving affection, praise, and attention
- Experience with success
- Personal definition of success or failure
- Response to negative feedback or criticism

Parents have a direct impact on the first two conditions that Coopersmith identified. For example, parents are a primary source of affection, praise, and attention—especially for younger adolescents. Additionally, parents structure situations that may help their children experience success. From this foundation of parent involvement, adolescents create an interpretation of success or failure and develop a response to feedback. Family relationships will be discussed further in a review of attachment (Chapter 5) and parenting style (Chapter 6). At this point, one should simply be sensitive to family influences on self-esteem. If an adolescent client has low self-esteem, one should assess family relationships and intervene at both the individual and family level.

PRESENTING PROBLEMS ASSOCIATED WITH SELF-ESTEEM

A variety of factors associated with self-esteem and clinical implications associated with these factors have been discussed. In some cases, self-esteem may have a hidden influence on the presenting problem. In this section the contribution of self-esteem to four areas: *school, family interaction, anti-social behavior,* and *suicide* are briefly reviewed.

School

Adolescents who have low self-esteem struggle academically and, perhaps because they are not doing well, are more likely to skip classes. Adolescents who have low self-esteem are also more likely to be isolated and withdrawn in the classroom. As a result, they are more likely to experience conflict with their teachers and peers. Parents may seek therapy for their adolescent because of poor grades, truancy, or problems associated with classroom behavior. Since self-esteem may have some influence on these presenting problems, we should take the time to conduct a thorough assessment of the adolescent's self-esteem as well as family dynamics.

What if it is discovered that the adolescent has low self-esteem? Because parent-adolescent interaction and parenting style influence self-esteem, an assessment of family factors should be conducted. (Assessment and intervention strategies associated with family dynamics will be discussed in Chapter 6.) If self-esteem is associated with academic performance, Susan Harter (1998) recommends a multipronged approach:

- Help the adolescent cultivate realistic expectations about performance.
- Encourage the adolescent to try new activities and cultivate situations that facilitate some level of success.
- Cultivate a support network—which would hopefully include parents but others as well—to help promote more positive regard.

Harter refers to this type of approach as a skill-based intervention and suggests that it is more useful than a "self-enhancement" approach. A self-enhancement approach is primarily concerned with helping an adolescent improve self-regard; improvement in school is seen as a result of improved self-esteem. Research seems to support Harter's conclusion, but therapy with the adolescent and the family could address both dimensions.

Family Interaction

Adolescents with low self-esteem are more likely to withdraw from their families and initiate more conflict with their parents and siblings. These adolescents may also experience problems at school or they may only act this way with family members. So, a family may initiate therapy because the child is a problem at school, at home, or in both settings. As before, assessment of self-esteem and family interaction should be a routine part of assessment.

Antisocial Behavior

Adolescents who have low self-esteem are more likely to abuse alcohol or other illegal substances, be sexually promiscuous, and engage in other risky behaviors. In each of these cases, the consequences of these behaviors are life threatening and safety should be a primary concern early in therapy. The extent to which low self-esteem may contribute to these problems should be examined.

Suicide

Darren Wozny will address suicide in Chapter 10. At this point, though, it is important to note that self-esteem is associated with suicide. Self-esteem, as previously discussed, is related to symptoms of depression. Depression, in turn, is associated with suicide. Two aspects of the relationship between self-esteem and depression need to be addressed. First, depression includes three dimensions: *self-worth, affect,* and *general hopelessness* (Harter, 1993), therefore assessment should address each of these dimensions. Second, these dimensions of depression are influenced by peer and parent support.

As with antisocial behavior, one's initial attention should be directed to safety issues. One who continues to work with an adolescent who has attempted suicide or who is at risk for attempting suicide should assess both dimensions of depression and self-esteem. To what extent does the adolescent experience feelings of support from friends and family? Which dimensions of depression seem the most salient for the particular client? Recall from Chapter 1 the case of Catherine, who was argumentative with her parents because she felt that her parents were intrusive. Catherine's parents initiated therapy with me because Catherine was rushed to the hospital after she swallowed a bottle of pills.

In Catherine's case, her parents were involved in her life and showed a distinct interest in her activities. This is consistent with Rosenberg's (1963, 1979) suggestion that parents should show interest in the lives of their children. Her parents also clearly communicated their expectations and set clear boundaries for Catherine; this was consistent with one of the family factors identified by Coopersmith (1967). As I worked with Catherine and her family, it seemed that other aspects associated with self-esteem were missing and that low self-esteem was associated with her suicide attempt. For example, although her parents were actively involved in Catherine's life, they did not clearly communicate acceptance of her. Additionally, Catherine did not experience her parents as respectful of her uniqueness and individuality.

In the early stages we focused on Catherine's safety. In time, I decided to focus on parental support. During a family session, Catherine complained that her parents were overbearing and did not trust her: "Mom searches through my stuff, eavesdrops on the phone, and checks up on me when I go out with my friends."

"Why do you think they do this?" I asked.

"Because they want to control me."

"Why else might they do these things?" I pressed.

"I don't know," Catherine replied.

Mable and Ben, Catherine's parents, confirmed that they did "spy" on Catherine because they were concerned about her. "What are you concerned about?" I asked.

"We're afraid that she'll get hurt."

"So do you do this because you care about what happens to your daughter?" I asked.

"Of course."

Catherine listened silently, looking down at her shoes. Her arms were folded tightly across her chest and the muscles in her jaw seemed tense. Noticing her body language, which suggested that Catherine was angry, I asked, "Is it hard for you to accept that your parents are legitimately concerned about you?"

"I think it's bullshit. I think they're both full of shit and that you're full of shit if you buy this. They don't give a damn about me."

This seemed to hit a nerve. Ben bristled and started to snap at her. "Don't you use that kind of language with me."

I moved to stop the argument. "Maybe I am full of shit, Catherine. But what if your parents really are concerned about you and they are trying to protect you? Would you feel differently if somehow you knew that your parents were doing these things because they were concerned about you?"

"Well, yeah. But I still don't believe them. They're just saying that to impress you."

"Maybe they are. Maybe they aren't. But let's pretend that somehow we knew beyond a shadow of a doubt that they did care about you. How would you feel? Instead of acting angry, how would you act?"

"I don't know," she answered. I was asking Catherine to switch her interpretation of her parent's behavior, so I wasn't surprised that she was having a hard time identifying a specific difference. I was encouraged, though, that she thought she would feel different if she somehow knew that her parents did care about her. I wanted to build on this idea, so I turned back to Mable and Ben.

"Okay, you're concerned that your daughter might get hurt. That suggests to me that you're responsible parents who are trying to protect their daughter. But can you see Catherine's side of this? Is it possible that your attempts to 'protect' Catherine are actually back-firing?"

"Maybe," Mable answered.

"I guess so," Ben replied.

"Well, that suggests that we need to find other ways for you to demonstrate to Catherine that you care about her." I looked at each member of the family and asked, "How else can you show Catherine that you care about her?" This began the process of cultivating supportive relationships in the family. The process was not always smooth. We had extended sessions in which parents and daughter yelled at one another and mutual mistrust seemed to be the norm. I continued to press for support. In time, the family began to yell less. As support increased, Catherine reported that she was feeling better about herself. In the three years following treatment, Catherine did not initiate any further attempts at suicide.

ASSESSMENT OF SELF-ESTEEM

At this point it should be apparent that assessment of self-esteem should be an important part of any therapy with adolescents. Self-esteem can be assessed clinically by paying attention to the language that clients use. To what extent does the client demonstrate self-acceptance? Are the self-references negative, positive, or neutral? What is the emotional response to evaluative statements? For example, a boy might say, "I suck at basketball" in a tone that suggests that he is angry or despondent. Or he could make the statement in a matter-of-fact tone that suggests that he is simply commenting on a skill that is of little importance to him.

Relevant Assessment Measures

At our clinic, all clients routinely receive a package of assessment instruments. Adolescent clients complete two scales that relate to self-esteem: the *Rosenberg Self-Esteem Scale* (Rosenberg, 1979) and, because family dynamics influence self-esteem, the *McMaster Family Assessment Device* (Epstein, Baldwin, and Bishop, 1983). Both of these scales are developmentally appropriate for adolescents. It may also be helpful to administer the Internal Control Index (Duttweiler, 1984), discussed later in this chapter, since self-esteem is associated with locus of control.

The Rosenberg Self-Esteem Scale, developed by the late Dr. Morris Rosenberg, is a ten-item scale that is developmentally appropriate for adolescents: it was originally designed for high school students. This scale measures the respondent's perception of global self-worth and research has demonstrated that it is a reliable, valid measure of self-esteem (Fischer and Corcoran, 1994).[1]

The McMaster Family Assessment Device is a sixty-item questionnaire designed to measure seven aspects of family functioning: (1) problem solving; (2) communication; (3) roles; (4) affective responsiveness; (5) affective involvement; (6) behavior control; and (7) general functioning (Epstein, Baldwin, and Bishop, 1983). The device is appropriate for adolescents in either concrete operations or formal operations stage. In evaluating influences on self-esteem, I am particularly interested in looking at the scores for communication, affective responsiveness (the degree to which family members respond emotionally to each other), and affective involvement (the degree to which family members are emotionally involved with each other). The McMaster Model of Family Functioning and this assessment device are discussed further in Chapter 6.

As mentioned in the introduction to this book, assessment is an ongoing process, and results from scales serve two purposes: (1) help us understand the client and prepare a treatment plan; (2) discuss findings with our clients. To discuss findings and to cultivate a better understanding about the influence of self-esteem or family dynamics, I often ask clients to talk further about their responses to specific questions. For example, I might ask a parent or adolescent to explain a response to the following item on the Family Assessment Device: "Some of us just don't respond emotionally" (Epstein, Baldwin, and Bishop, 1983). Depending on the response, I might ask, "How do you think that this kind of emotional responding is related to your sense of self-worth?"

LOCUS OF CONTROL

Locus of control refers to one's belief about the ability to control one's own life. Morris Rosenberg, who has investigated the relationship between self-esteem and locus of control, describes the difference between an *internal locus of control* and an *external locus of control.* "People characterized by an internal locus of control felt that what happened to them in life was essentially a consequence of their own actions. Those with an external locus of control orientation tended to feel that what happened to them was a consequence of events governed by external forces" (Rosenberg, 1985, p. 224). Rosenberg summarized research findings on the significance of locus of control:

- Children and adolescents who have an external locus of control have lower self-esteem. They also show more symptoms of depression, anxiety, impulsivity, irritability, resentment, and alienation.
- Children and adolescents who have an internal locus of control earn better grades in school. They are also happier and more satisfied with their lives.

Developmentally, Rosenberg reports that internal locus of control increases with age. This suggests that early adolescents are particularly vulnerable to problems associated with an external locus of control, so assessment should be routinely completed for younger adolescents. It also suggests that when working with older adolescents who exhibit depression, anxiety, irritability, resentment, or alienation, locus of control should be assessed. In either case, one would seek to enhance an internal locus of control.

Influences on Locus of Control

In his book *Social and Personality Development*, William Damon reports that locus of control is influenced by responsiveness of interpersonal relationships with significant others as well as economic status of the child's family. Lack of responsiveness on the part of significant others seems to have a substantial influence on locus of control. "Parental indifference, peer hostility, the impersonality of school, all may confront children with examples of unpleasant events that they cannot control" (Damon, 1983, pp. 229-230). Damon discusses intervention:

- *Assess parent style of providing feedback.* "Suggestive" styles of parenting interactions are associated with internal locus of control. Example: "Why don't you try to do it this way?" versus "Do it like this."
- *Help adolescents identify their contribution to failure and help parents provide specific feedback.* In an experimental study, children who were given specific feedback about failure on math problems did better on subsequent problems than children who were simply told that they did not do well. Children who were not given specific feedback became apathetic and lost interest in doing additional problems. In addition to helping identify their own contributions, parents could be encouraged to provide specific feedback rather than global evaluations.
- *Assess attitude and feedback styles of teachers.* Research suggests that teachers are more likely to hold the belief that girls who are unable to solve a problem are incompetent while boys who are unable to solve a problem are not trying hard enough. As a result, boys receive feedback from teachers that encourages them to continue to solve problems while girls receive feedback associated with giving up. Damon concludes: "[W]e could connect this differential treatment of the sexes with the far greater incidence of perceived helplessness and depression found in women at all ages" (1983, p. 230). Thus, one would want to inquire about classroom management, especially if girls are demonstrating an external locus of control. In these cases, encourage parents to initiate a parent-teacher conference to discuss the problem.

Locus of control is also influenced by factors that influence opportunities available to the family. For example, children who live in poverty are more likely to demonstrate external locus of control because opportunities available to the child and the family are limited. In these cases, day-to-day life is very much influenced by external sources (e.g., unemployment; availability of affordable housing or child care). Therapists should be sensitive, then, to external conditions that affect the lives of their clients so that clinical intervention reflects these conditions.

Locus of Control Assessment

The Internal Control Index (Duttweiler, 1984) is a twenty-eight-item instrument designed to measure expectations about reinforcement. Clients who expect encouragement and reinforcement from others as a source of motivation demonstrate an external locus of control. The following question from the Internal Control Index exemplifies this expectation: "I need someone else to praise my work before I am satisfied with what I've done." In contrast, an internal locus of control would be demonstrated by positive responses to an item such as the following: "Whenever something good happens to me, I feel it is because I've earned it." Research suggests that the validity and reliability for this scale are suitable for clinical assessment.[2]

SUMMARY

Self-esteem is another important aspect of adolescent development that influences presenting problems that range from academic difficulty to suicide. It seems to be influenced by perception of peer and family support as well as locus of control, so assessment and intervention should address each.

SECTION II:
INTERPERSONAL RELATIONSHIPS

Chapter 5

Attachment

Attachment is one of the most important aspsects of the developmental-systemic model. John Byng-Hall is a family therapist who serves as a consultant on child and adolescent psychiatry at the Tavistock Clinic in London. He has published a number of articles and chapters suggesting that attachment theory and research make a significant contribution to understanding families and family therapy process. For example, research based on attachment theory is consistent with propositions from Bowenian, structural, object relations, and narrative therapies. Byng-Hall suggests that the attachment literature can be used to supplement traditional models of family therapy: "Attachments lie at the heart of family life. They create bonds that can provide care and protection across the life cycle (Ainsworth, 1991), and can evoke the most intense emotions—joy in the making, anguish in the breaking—or create problems if they become insecure" (Byng-Hall, 1995, p. 45).

Larry, a seventeen-year-old, seems to have a close relationship with his mother, Mary, and an antagonistic one with her third husband, Rick. In contrast, Lance, who is also seventeen years old, seems to have a better relationship with his stepfather than with his biological mother. Lynn, a single mother, seems exasperated that Mindy, her thirteen-year-old daughter, seems to "take out her frustrations with her father on me and her sisters." In each of these cases, the bond between an adolescent and her or his parents seems to affect family dynamics. It may be helpful to understand these bonds by reviewing *attachment,* a significant aspect of parent-child relationships that developmental and social psychologists have extensively investigated.

Attachment seems to be a misunderstood concept that has not received adequate attention in the family therapy literature. Perhaps

misunderstandings about attachment have impaired its incorpora-
tion into mainstream family therapy. Aspects of attachment, types
of attachment in children and adults, its significance in families
with adolescents, and family therapy implications will be reviewed.

First, though, some misperceptions about attachment should be
cleared up. Like other psychological constructs such as egocentrism
and self-esteem, attachment is used in common language to refer
primarily to a bond between parents, typically mothers, and their
children. Casual use of the term seems to confuse attachment with
the process of *imprinting* to suggest that it can only develop shortly
after birth. Conrad Lorenz provided a dramatic and widely known
example of the imprinting process. He created a situation in which
newborn chicks interacted only with him shortly after birth. Due to
this interaction, the chicks responded to Lorenz as if he were their
mother. For example, they followed him in a single-file line as they
would their mother when he took a walk.

Also, a distraught mother once expressed fear that she would
never be able to bond with her premature daughter because the
newborn was placed in an incubator. Similarly, parents who adopt
children often wonder if they will be able to cultivate an appropriate
attachment. In the remainder of this chapter, these misconceptions
and clinical implications of attachment will be addressed.

WHAT IS ATTACHMENT?

John Bowlby and Mary Ainsworth are the two pioneers in the
area of attachment. John Byng-Hall suggested that Bowlby wrote
one of the first manuscripts about family therapy in 1949. According
to Byng-Hall, Bowlby was a "steadfast supporter of family therapy"
(Byng-Hall, 1999, p. 625, based on Byng-Hall, 1991). Bowlby
suggested that attachment with an adult caregiver ensured the safety
of children.

Jude Cassidy recently provided a succinct yet thorough overview
of attachment theory. According to Cassidy, Bowlby distinguished
between three aspects of attachment: (1) *attachment behavior,*
(2) *attachment behavioral system,* and (3) *attachment bond.* The
first, attachment behavior, refers to actions that promote proximity
to an attachment figure. Children make eye contact, cry, or make

gestures as methods to engage their parents. Attachment behavioral system refers to a particular repertoire of behaviors that an individual uses. Attachment bond refers to an affectional tie: "this bond is not between two people; it is instead a bond that one individual has to another individual who is perceived as stronger and wiser. . . . A person can be attached to a person who is not in turn attached to him or her" (Cassidy, 1999, p. 12). Cassidy reported several important propositions about attachment theory:

1. The attachment bond is only one feature of a parent-child relationship. Caregivers also serve as playmates, teachers, and disciplinarians.
2. A child may demonstrate attachment behavior with someone for whom they do not share an attachment bond.
3. Children experience multiple attachments but the quality of the attachment bond is not the same in each relationship. The quality of the bond is influenced by amount of interaction, quality of care provided, and emotional investment of the caregiver.

The third proposition was exemplified in the three brief descriptions of parent-adolescent relationships presented at the beginning of this chapter: each of the adolescents seemed to demonstrate a different type of attachment relationship with caregivers. These cases will be explored further as aspects of attachment are discussed.

Behavioral Systems

The following material is based on Cassidy's (1999) review. Bowlby suggested that an attachment behavioral system served an evolutionary function because it encouraged protection of children who are dependent on adults for safety. Bowlby also suggested that two other behavioral systems interact with the attachment behavioral system. First, the *exploratory behavioral system* promotes survival because curiosity helps children learn about and adapt to their environment. This system reduces attachment behavior. Second, the *fear behavioral system* promotes safety and, as a result, engages the attachment system.

Larry, a young man briefly mentioned in the introduction to this chapter, seemed to demonstrate the importance of both of these behavioral systems. He reported that he missed both his biological father and his mother's second husband, especially the second husband, whom he remembered fondly. After his mother divorced her second husband, Larry saw very little of him. Now that his mother had remarried, Larry seemed reluctant to explore a relationship with her new husband, Rick. This suggests that the fear behavioral system was interfering with the exploratory behavioral system: Larry seemed afraid to cultivate a relationship (exploratory behavioral system) with Rick for fear that Rick and his mother might divorce. This seemed to interfere with processes associated with the attachment behavioral system.

TYPES OF ATTACHMENT

Research has systematically examined attachment style in children and seems to support the categories for styles of attachment that have been developed. Development of a particular attachment style seems influenced by dynamics of the caregiver-child relationship. Research on attachment in children has inspired research on adult attachment. Byng-Hall (1999) suggests that the attachment styles of both parents and children influences the family system. In this section, types of attachment in children and adults are reviewed, and the ways in which they interact are discussed. In the following section, the significance of attachment in adolescence will be discussed.

Types of Attachment in Children

Mary Ainsworth noticed that children frequently interrupted play behavior to literally touch base with their caregiver before returning to play. Ainsworth suspected that this behavior represented the interconnectedness between the exploratory and attachment behavioral systems. Ainsworth developed the Strange Situation (SS) test to evaluate types of attachment (Ainsworth, Waters, and Wall, 1978); assessment of attachment style was also based on observation of children in their home environment. Through the SS, Ainsworth examined the response of children to a strange situation:

children in her laboratory (the strange situation) were briefly separated from their parents twice, once for three minutes and once for six minutes. Behaviors of the parents and children were observed prior to separation and after each separation. Four styles of attachment have been developed based on research using the SS test: *secure, avoidant, resistant or ambivalent,* and *disorganized/disoriented* (Ainsworth, Waters, and Wall, 1978; Main and Solomon, 1990). Material about the first three categories is based on the work of Mary Ainsworth and her colleagues. The material about the final category is based on the work of Main and Solomon.

Secure Attachment

Most children in the general population (estimates range from 50 to 75 percent) can be classified as securely attached. During the SS test, the child explores the room prior to separation and shows distress when the caregiver leaves. When they are reunited, both the caregiver and the child seem pleased to see each other and begin to interact. Home observation identified the following characteristics associated with parent-child interactions:

- Communication between caregiver and child seems to be warm and sensitive. Child does not seem afraid to express anger.
- Caregiver permits age-appropriate autonomy and exploration. There is flexibility in proximity: child and caregiver operate independently and touch base with each other from time to time.
- Caregiver seems to have a coherent view of attachment and recognizes that it is important to the child.
- Caregiver and child seem to have fun interacting.

Avoidant Attachment

In the general population, 15 to 30 percent of children can be classified as avoidant. During the SS test, the child continues to explore the room after separation showing limited, if any, distress. When the caregiver returns, the child turns away from the caregiver and moves toward a toy in the room. The caregiver pays more attention to objects in the room than the child. If the child is picked up by the caregiver, he or she makes motions to be put down. Although behaviors suggest that these children are unaffected by the separation, research suggests that they remain aroused much longer than securely attached children: the avoidant child continues to show physiological signs of anxiety. The strategy to withdraw from the caregiver despite physiological arousal suggests that the child is attempting to deactivate feelings of insecurity by focusing on other objects. Home observation identified the following characteristics associated with parent-child interactions:

- Caregiver seems to respond negatively to the child's attempts to make contact: the caregiver withdraws when the child is sad.
- Caregiver seems to demonstrate more rejecting behaviors toward child.
- Child demonstrates more anger at home than in the lab setting.
- Play behavior seems to serve as a distraction from attachment needs.

Resistant or Ambivalent Attachment

Byng-Hall (1995) has suggested that resistant or ambivalent relationships are similar to enmeshed relationships. The child seems to cling to caregivers because of experiences in which the caregiver is intermittently unavailable (Byng-Hall, 1995). In the general population, from 4 to 25 percent can be classified as resistant or ambivalent. During the SS test, the child appears to be distressed prior to the two separations and seems preoccupied with the caregiver throughout the procedure. The child does not seem to be soothed by the presence of the caregiver and may appear angry or passive. The child is unlikely to return to exploration after a reunion. Home observation identified the following characteristics associated with parent-child interactions:

- Caregiver seems committed to the task of nurturing but is often emotionally unavailable.
- The child seems to have learned that the caregiver is capable of responding if he or she is persistent at seeking attention, so the child stays in close proximity to the caregiver.

• Some children may take care of their parents as a way to foster interaction. This may, according to Byng-Hall (1995), contribute to parentification of children.

Disorganized/Disoriented Attachment

In the general population, 15 to 25 percent of children can be classified as disorganized/disoriented. Research suggests that a significant number of children (as many as 80 percent) who are maltreated can be classified in this category. Main and Solomon (1990), in coding videotapes of the SS test, experienced difficulty classifying all children using the previous three categories because some children did not respond systematically to the reunion part of the experience. In the presence of caregivers, these children may (1) freeze with a trancelike expression, (2) rise when caregivers enter the room, (3) fall to the floor, or (4) cling to caregiver while leaning away from caregiver. Their other behaviors could be classified into one of the other categories. Observations of these children at home suggest that the idiosyncratic response to the SS test may be related to the way they avoid abuse at home. For example, children who cower on the floor in the SS test may have cultivated this cowering behavior as a way to protect themselves from injury.

Types of Attachment in Adults

Research on attachment styles in children inspired investigation of attachment styles in adults. An Adult Attachment Interview (AAI) (George, Kaplan, and Main, 1984) was developed to assess attachment styles in adults and has been revised three times. During the AAI, the participants are asked to provide five adjectives that describe each parent and an example of an episode that illustrates each adjective. Interviewers inquire about the following: (a) how caregivers responded to the participant when he or she was upset; (b) whether caregivers threatened him or her; (c) whether he or she felt rejected by caregivers; (d) explanation for caregivers' behavior; and (e) effect of these childhood experiences on the participant's adult personality. The attachment of the participant's children can be predicted from these interviews. The responses are evaluated on two dimensions.

The first dimension is *coherence.* Coherence refers to answers that (1) provide a clear and convincing description; (2) are truthful, succinct, and complete; and (3) are presented in a clear and orderly manner. The second dimension is the *ability to reflect on the motives of others.* Four types of adult attachment have been identified: *secure/autonomous, dismissing, preoccupied,* and *unresolved/disorganized.* We will rely on the work of Main, Kaplan, and Cassidy (1985) and Byng-Hall (1995) to describe these important categories.

Secure/Autonomous Adult Attachment

Research using the AAI suggests that caregivers seem to be able to respond appropriately to children if they can make sense of their own childhood experience and are able to understand the motives of others. This seems to facilitate secure attachment in their children. As a caregiver, the person seems to recognize that attachment is important.

Dismissing Adult Attachment

Responses on the AAI are not coherent: adjectives used to describe caregivers are usually positive but descriptions either do not support the positive adjective or actively contradict it. The person seems to be dismissive about the importance of attachment. This type of adult attachment promotes avoidant attachment in children. "The shared parent/child attachment strategy is to maintain distance . . . in order to reduce the likelihood of emotional outbursts that might lead to rejections. The price is a loss of sensitive care for the child when it is needed" (Byng-Hall, 1995, p. 50).

Preoccupied Adult Attachment

Responses on the AAI are not coherent: descriptions of adjectives include vague references. The person seems to be preoccupied with past relationship experiences and may appear angry. As a result, boundaries in the family become blurred. This type of adult attachment promotes resistant or ambivalent attachment in children. "There is a great deal of mutual monitoring and mind reading, all in an attempt to forestall any potential drifting away on the part of either the parent or the child" (Byng-Hall, 1995, p. 50).

Unresolved/Disorganized Adult Attachment

This person seems frightened by the memory of past trauma, which may promote momentary disassociation. Responses on the AAI about topics that deal with loss or abuse are incoherent. For example, the person might use language suggesting that someone who is deceased is still alive. Other responses are consistent with the other categories. This type of adult attachment promotes disorganized/disoriented attachment in children. "The general impression is that the parent does not have the child in mind at all but, rather, is scripting the child into some past drama. . . . As the children grow older, overall strategies do seem to evolve. They either become more controlling of the parent, often in a punitive way, or they become caretaking of their parents" (Byng-Hall, 1995, p. 51).

ATTACHMENT IN ADOLESCENCE

Based on their review of research on attachment in adolescence, Joseph P. Allen and Deborah Land suggest that adolescents are motivated to become less dependent on their parents during this transitional period. This is not to say that parents are unimportant. The task for adolescents, Allen and Land (1999) suggest, is to develop a relationship with their parents that is more mutual. They concluded that "research is increasingly showing that adolescent autonomy is most easily established not at the expense of attachment relationships with parents but against a backdrop of secure relationships that are likely to endure well beyond adolescence" (p. 319). Allen and Land continue:

> From this perspective, adolescence is not a period in which attachment needs and behaviors are relinquished; rather, it is one in which they are gradually transferred to peers. This transfer also involves a *transformation* from hierarchical attachment relationships (in which one primarily receives care

from a caregiver) to peer attachment relationships (in which one both receives and offers care and support). (1999, p. 323)

Attachment relationships in adolescence are influenced by cognitive development. For example, adolescents who demonstrate formal operational thinking—particularly the capacity for abstract thought—are able to develop a more "overarching" view of attachment relationships (Allen and Land, 1999). Additionally, increases in differentiation of self transform attachment relationships so that they "become more internally based and less centered around a particular relationship" (Allen and Land, 1999, p. 320). These two transitions suggest that attachment relationships continue to be important during adolescence.

Allen and Land suggest that secure attachment in adolescents will promote family functioning. For example, according to a study by Cathron L. Hilburn Cobb (1996), a secure attachment to *both* parents contributes to a family environment that features high collaboration and high exploration. Insecure attachment in adolescents, however, may create problems in families for three reasons:

1. Caregivers may interpret individuation efforts as a threat to their relationship with their adolescent child.
2. Insecurely attached adolescents and their parents may become overwhelmed by affect associated with individuation which, in turn, contributes to conflict.
3. Insecurely attached adolescents may become easily frustrated because they do not expect to be heard or understood by a parent.

For Lance, the seventeen-year-old who seemed to have a better relationship with his stepfather Dave than his biological mother Ann and his family, all of these factors seemed to contribute to family conflict. Ann described Lance as a "smart ass" and Dave suggested that Lance was "disrespectful to his mother. We [Lance and Dave] have a good relationship but the boy needs to learn how to treat his mother better. He needs to show her more respect. He treats her like a dog." Everyone claimed that Lance had always had a better relationship with Dave than Ann, but the intense conflict in the family was a recent phenomenon.

"You said that your problems have 'gotten out of hand' in the past year. What has been happening?" I asked.

Dave replied quickly. "Lance has gotten uppity. He seems to think that he can boss his mother around and make his own rules."

I wondered if the recent conflict was associated with individuation (e.g., Lance's desire to "make his own rules") as well as long-simmering difficulties associated with attachment. I further wondered if Lance, who seemed to be insecurely attached to his mother, was acting out of that frustration because he did not expect to be understood by her. Although I wondered about these two features of the relationship, I did not inquire about the attachment bond between Lance and Ann. Rather, I took a solution-focused approach and asked questions about the bond between Lance and Dave, and I stayed on the topic of respect since it was important to Ann and Dave.

"Why do you think that Lance is more respectful to you than Ann?" I asked. "Are you more likely to punish him if he's disrespectful? Does he treat her badly because he can get away with it? Why is there this difference?"

Ann replied this time. "No, I'm not a pushover. I'm the disciplinarian. If any of the kids get in trouble, they know that I'll get after them."

"Okay. So, Ann's the disciplinarian in the family. Now we know that Lance knows how to be respectful because you've said that he treats only Ann disrespectfully. So I guess I'm wondering about the relationship between Lance and Dave. Lance, what is it about your relationship with Dave that you interact with him differently than your mom?"

"I dunno," he replied. Dave started to speak but I said that I wanted to hear Lance's answer. I asked again, "What's different, Lance?"

"I dunno. I guess I can count on Dave. He listens to me. He's not always telling me that I'm stupid. We do things together." This seemed to be important information that confirmed Cobb's research: Lance's response suggested that he could not depend on his mother and, now that he was in the process of individuating, he seemed more vocal about expressing his frustration.

ATTACHMENT IN FAMILIES

Family As a Secure Base

From a family systems perspective, Byng-Hall (1995, 1999) suggests that the family contributes to attachment by providing a *secure family base*, defined as "a family that provides a reliable and readily available network of attachment relationships, and appropriate caregivers, from which all members of the family are able to feel sufficiently secure to explore their potential" (p. 627). Byng-Hall suggests that two factors are associated with a secure family base. First, he suggests that there is a shared awareness that attachment relationships are important and care for others is a priority in the family. Second, he contends that family members should support one another in providing care for each other. Byng-Hall (1995, 1999) has also identified factors that undermine a secure family base.

1. Fear of losing an attachment figure or actual loss of an attachment figure.
2. A child clings to one caregiver and rejects relationships with other caregivers. Byng-Hall refers to this as "capturing" an attachment figure.
3. Turning to an inappropriate attachment figure (e.g., if one parent is not supporting the other parent, a child may be used as an attachment figure).
4. Conflict within relationships, particularly abusive relationships.
5. Negative self-fulfilling prophecies: there is an expectation that losses from other generations will be repeated.

Influence of Attachment on Distance Regulation in Families

Distance regulation is a common theme in many models of family therapy. For example, structural therapy suggests that there are problems associated with relationships that are too close (enmeshed) or too distant (disengaged). Similarly, Murray Bowen (1985) suggested that families should include some level of differentiation between members. Byng-Hall (1995, 1999) suggests that attachment relationships contribute to problematic distance regulation in families.

FAMILY THERAPY IMPLICATIONS

In this chapter, the focus has been on the value of attachment theory in adolescence, and important dimensions of attachment have been reviewed. Parenting issues that affect attachment will be addressed in the following chapter on parenting. Before ending this chapter, implications of attachment theory for family therapy and strategies for assessing attachment in our work with adolescents and their families will be discussed.

Tasks in Therapy

Based on Bowlby, Byng-Hall (1995, 1999) identified four tasks for the family therapist to perform. Each of the tasks can be addressed from any number of approaches to family therapy.

Provide a Secure Therapeutic Base for the Family

This is similar to the idea in object relations family therapy of developing a "safe container" for therapy. Byng-Hall suggests that the therapist will serve as an attachment figure to family members. As a result, therapists should be regularly available to their clients throughout the clinical experience, and therapists should communicate their future availability.

Work with Current Significant Relationships

Byng-Hall (1995) suggests that it may be helpful to normalize difficulties associated with attachment. "Using knowledge of insecure attachment dynamics, therapists can positively connote behavior that would otherwise appear to be merely hostile, distancing, or controlling" (pp. 54-55). In his later chapter, Byng-Hall (1999) elaborates:

> Attachment theory can offer explanations that are clear to both therapist and family, and that make sense out of what may be otherwise perplexing. For instance, a child who is angry, demanding, and controlling is often seen as intentionally bad, but

the child can be seen in a different light if described as insecure and trying to make sure he or she is in the parents' minds
when he or she feels unloved and unlovable. (p. 636)

This approach seemed to help Lynn and Mindy. Recall that Lynn,
who is a single mother, reported that Mindy "took out her frustrations with her father on me and her sisters." I asked about differences in the relationships and Mindy reported that she thought she
had a much stronger relationship with her mother than her father.
"Is it possible that you become angry with your mother because you
know that she won't push you away?" I asked.

"I guess so," Mindy replied. "Dad's kind of moody and if you
piss him off he won't call for weeks." This exemplified, as did other
cases in this chapter, that adolescents have multiple attachment
relationships. In this case, Mindy seemed to have a secure attachment to her mother, so it was safer for her to express anger at her
mother than her father. This explanation helped Lynn understand
her daughter's behavior so that she could respond with compassion.

In addition to providing reframes, Byng-Hall contends that we
should attend to significant relationships by promoting more coherent narratives for the family. Narrative therapy techniques would
be particularly helpful. Two other types of problems that relate to
current significant relationships may require attention: distance
conflicts and power battles. Structural techniques may be helpful
for those problems.

Explore the Relationship Between Family Members and the Therapist

Because therapists become part of the family system during therapy, therapists should pay attention to their influence. "Feeling understood is crucial to family members' establishing secure attachments
to the therapist" (Byng-Hall, 1999, p. 636). Since therapists may be
seen as attachment figures, an experiential approach to therapy may
help address these issues. Augustus Napier and Carl Whitaker's *The
Family Crucible* (1978) should be mandatory reading for therapists
interested in incorporating attachment theory into their clinical work.

Review and Evaluate Ways in Which Current Relationship Patterns Are Influenced by Past Experiences

"Exploring the connections between stories of what happened in past generations and what is happening now in the session can help the therapist and the family members to elucidate what comes from the past, and then to assess whether or not behaving in old ways is helpful now" (Byng-Hall, 1999, p. 639). This is similar to Murray Bowen's recommendation to "embrace" family history in order to promote differentiation. Narrative and symbolic experiential therapies could be used to help evaluate relationship patterns.

ASSESSMENT OF ATTACHMENT IN FAMILY THERAPY

To this point, the significance of attachment theory to adolescents has been addressed, attachment theory has been reviewed, and intervention strategies in family therapy with adolescents have been discussed. Before concluding this chapter, two methods to assess attachment in families are briefly discussed.

Self-Report Measures

Recent research suggests that measures of attachment should be reported as continuous dimensions rather than as fixed categories (e.g., secure, avoidant, anxious, disorganized). Gay C. Armsden and Mark T. Greenberg developed the Inventory of Parent and Peer Attachment (IPPA) (Armsden and Greenberg, 1987), a self-report measure of attachment for adolescents that is both exceptionally reliable and valid. The IPPA includes three twenty-five-item scales that measure attachment to mothers, fathers, and close friends. The IPPA uses subscales rather than classification categories. Three subscales measure important dimensions of attachment: trust, communication, and alienation.[1]

Clinical Assessment

John Byng-Hall (1995) developed the Family Separation Test to assess attachment during a family therapy session. It is very similar to Ainsworth's Strange Situation test. Parents are asked to leave the room when the therapist makes a particular signal. The parents remain out of the room for six minutes and the children remain in the room with the therapist. Upon their return, parents are asked to initially open the door and stand next to each other in the doorway for five seconds. They then are instructed to react naturally. Byng-Hall suggests that this provides clinical information about the following:

1. Difficulties associated with separation
2. Attachment behavior between siblings during the separation
3. Attachments to the therapist
4. Identification of parent preferences for each child
5. Clues about the nature of attachments in the family

SUMMARY

In this chapter, I have identified aspects of attachment, emphasized that children have multiple attachment relationships, and have suggested, following the recommendations of John Byng-Hall, that families serve as a secure base for adolescents. I also discussed the importance of therapeutic relationship and reviewed tasks of therapy that can help facilitate attachment. These tasks suggest that therapy is as much about the quality of the relationship between therapist and family members as it is about clinical interventions. The following chapter will address aspects of parenting that influence attachment.

Chapter 6

Parent-Adolescent Relationship

Within the developmental-systemic model, family relationships—especially the parent-child relationship—are seen as significant influences. The importance of the parent-adolescent relationship has been discussed throughout this book. For example, it has been noted that parent support influences self-esteem and depression, which, in turn, influences suicidal ideation. The influence of parents on identity development and emotional development has also been examined. The influence of parents on peer relationships, sexuality, and substance abuse will be examined in the following chapters. In the previous chapter, I discussed the work of John Byng-Hall, who suggested attachment is the result of relationships with caregivers and other family members. He proposed that family relationships contribute to a secure family base for attachment. The present chapter builds on material that was reviewed in the previous chapter by focusing on aspects of parenting that influence attachment, including factors associated with parental influence, a conceptualization of "healthy" family functioning, parenting styles, and parenting practices.

Often, families initiate therapy with adolescents because of a particular problem (e.g., substance abuse, academic difficulty) and some models of therapy might focus primarily on eliminating the "problem." Philip A. Cowan, Douglas Powell, and Carolyn Pape Cowan have developed a family systems perspective of parenting interventions that emphasizes broader goals that are consistent with facilitating attachment. This perspective provides a useful approach for conceptualizing family therapy with adolescents. Cowan, Powell, and Cowan (1998) suggest that the central task of parenting is "not simply [for parents] to keep their infants alive or provide appropriate discipline but to create the conditions in which children can develop to their fullest capacity both inside and outside the family" (p. 5). This suggests that therapy goals should focus on enhancing family relationships.

CONNECTEDNESS FOR ADOLESCENTS

Recall that there is a transition in attachment relationships during adolescence. Adolescents transfer their dependence for attachment from parents to peers, and attachment relationships in general become more mutual. Connectedness is a sign of mutuality that seems to influence attachment relationships. W. Andrew Collins and Daniel J. Repinski (1994) suggest that connectedness for adolescents is influenced by five factors: *trust, intimacy, closeness, positive affect,* and *communication.* The following review of these dimensions is based on Collins and Repinski (1994).[1]

Trust

Trust is a subjective experience. During adolescence, trust seems to be enhanced by communication in relationships and reduced by feelings of alienation and isolation. Mutual trust seems to develop in relationships in which there is a reciprocal pattern of cooperation. Developmentally, adolescents' experience of trust "becomes more differentiated and sophisticated in accord with developing cognitive abilities and an expanded repertoire of experience" (Collins and Repinski, 1994, p. 21).

Closeness and Intimacy

Intimacy and closeness are overlapping constructs, so these two dimensions are reviewed together. Intimacy refers to relationships in which "partners experience and express feelings, communicate verbally and nonverbally, satisfy social motives, augment or reduce social fears, talk and learn about themselves and their unique characteristics, and become 'close'" (Reiss and Shaver, 1988, p. 387, quoted in Collins and Repinski, 1994, p. 21). Intimacy seems to have two dimensions: (1) emotional communication and (2) validation. There seem to be developmental differences in the perception of intimacy between early and late adolescents. Younger adolescents seem to emphasize disclosure or personal thoughts and feelings while older adolescents seem to focus on feeling accepted and understood. Strategies to improve intimacy in families were reviewed when emotion was discussed in Chapter 2.

Positive Affect

Physical changes associated with puberty seem to be associated with less positive affect and more negative affect in families. The negative affect promotes increased stress, hurt feelings, and embarrassment. This point will be disscussed further in this chapter when the McMaster Model of Family Functioning is reviewed.

Communication

Communication is the process of exchanging information. Adolescents generally report that they are more satisfied with communication with mothers, who are perceived as more available, than fathers. This dimension will also be discussed further in a review of the McMaster Model of Family Functioning.

FUNCTIONS OF FAMILIES

Inge Seiffge-Krenke and Shmuel Shulman (1993) completed a review of research on stress, coping, and relationships in adolescence. Based on their review, they conclude that the best predictors of adolescent well-being are (1) the adolescent's perception of family cohesion and (2) an index of family stress. We will elaborate on each of these points.

The McMaster Model of Family Functioning

Nathan Epstein, Duane Bishop, and colleagues developed the McMaster Model of Family Functioning (Epstein et al., 1993), which has inspired a corresponding research instrument, the Family Assessment Device (FAD). Two subscales from the FAD were briefly discussed in the chapter on self-esteem (Chapter 4). The

McMaster model describes structural, occupational, and transactional properties of families and identifies six dimensions of family functioning: *problem solving, communication, roles, affective responsiveness, affective involvement, and behavior control.* Research suggests that these dimensions are associated with positive emotional health of adolescents (Westley and Epstein, 1969).

Problem Solving

Problem solving refers to the ability to resolve problems at a level that maintains effective family functioning (e.g., trying to think of different ways to solve problems). Problem solving influences attachment because if daily problems are not solved, the family seems to have less time to devote to nurturing and supportive relationships. According to the McMaster model, problem solving occurs in a seven-step sequence. If families experience difficulty in this area, it may be helpful to evaluate their approach to problem solving in order to identify stages in the sequence that might provide a particular challenge to the family. Epstein and his colleagues (1993) identify the following stages:

1. Identify the problem.
2. Communicate with appropriate people about the problem.
3. Develop a list of possible solutions.
4. Decide to implement one of the choices.
5. Carry out actions required to implement the choice.
6. Ensure that the task is completed.
7. Evaluate the effectiveness of the problem-solving process.

Communication

Communication refers to an exchange of information that enhances attachment behavior and attachment bond. Family members exchange information that is both factual and emotional, and communication is both verbal and nonverbal. Clinically, one would evaluate family messages for clarity, respect, direction, and intent. Four patterns of communication are described: *clear and direct, clear and indirect, unclear and direct,* and *unclear and indirect.*[2] If communication is not clear and direct, particular communication strategies may need to be addressed.

Roles

Family roles "are defined as the repetitive patterns of behavior by which family members fulfill family functions" (Epstein et al., 1993, p. 147). Megan Murphy and I addressed family functions in *The Encyclopedia of Parenting Theory and Research:*

> Instrumental functions are task-oriented duties in which someone represents the family to the outside world, usually through employment. Expressive functions are also referred to as socioemotional roles which include emotional labor such as nurturance and support. Children need to have both instrumental and expressive needs met; furthermore, they benefit from learning to complete both functions. Parents can facilitate this process by providing direct instruction and serving as role models. (Werner-Wilson and Murphy, 1999, p. 234)

Research suggests that (1) instrumental and emotional functions are important, and (2) flexible roles (e.g., mothers and fathers both provide nurturing) increase the likelihood that needs will be met (Werner-Wilson and Murphy, 1999). The first point is consistent with attachment theory and suggests that we would want to assess the extent to which emotional needs of family members are being met.

Affective Responsiveness

Affective responsiveness refers to "the ability to respond to a given stimulus with the appropriate quality and quantity of feelings: assesses individual family member's ability to experience appropriate emotional responses for a range of experiences" (Epstein et al., 1993, p. 149). Secure attachment is associated with caregivers who respond emotionally to children and also tolerate age-appropriate exploration. Problems with affective responsiveness are associated with emotional overinvolvement (enmeshment) or underinvolvement (disengagement).

Affective Involvement

This refers to the extent to which family members are interested in and place value on one another's activities and concerns. Epstein and colleagues (1993) identify six types of involvement:

1. Lack of involvement: no interest or investment in one another
2. Involvement without feeling: interest is primarily intellectual in nature
3. Narcissistic involvement: interest in others only occurs if there is a personal benefit
4. Empathic involvement: interest in others for the sake of the others
5. Overinvolvement: excessive interest and intrusiveness
6. Symbiotic involvement: extreme and pathological interest in others

Attachment relationships are enhanced by empathy, so the therapist should help family members recognize and respect the experiences of other family members.

Behavior Control

This refers to family rules that influence meeting the needs of family members in three areas: protection from physical danger, fulfillment of psychobiological needs (e.g., food, shelter, physical interaction), and fulfillment of interpersonal needs. "We are interested in the standards or rules the family sets in these areas and in the latitude they allow around the standard" (Epstein et al., 1993, p. 152). Rigid rules are likely to interfere with attachment relationships.

Clinical Assessment of Family Functioning

The McMaster Family Assessment Device (FAD) (Epstein, Baldwin, and Bishop, 1983) is a sixty-item questionnaire that includes a subscale for each of the six dimensions described in the model. It also includes a score for general functioning. It is appropriate for adolescents in either concrete operations or formal operations and has high reliability and validity.[3]

Stress and Family Support

As discussed, the nature of the parent-adolescent relationship changes. These changes are stressful for both the parent and the adolescent (Kirchler, Palmonari, and Pombeni, 1993). Thomas Ashby Wills, Elaine A. Blechman, and Grace McNamara (1996) reviewed the interaction between family support and adolescent coping. Their description of supportive families is consistent with the dimensions described in the McMaster Model of Family Functioning. They proposed that effective communication would be perceived as support by adolescents and would promote competence through the following processes (Wills, Blechman, and McNamara, 1996):

1. Emotional support in families increases self-esteem and feelings of validation.
2. Emotional support in families increases the probability that adolescents will seek out family members to help cope with problems with school and friends.
3. Adolescents who experience family support are more likely to be active in the community.

PARENTAL INFLUENCE

In the chapter on attachment (Chapter 5), it was noted that peer influence is mediated by the quality of the parent-adolescent relationship. William Damon summarized research on parental influence:

Most empirical research has found that adolescents generally are attached to their home life in a strong and positive way. The large majority of adolescents find their family situation happy and harmonious. Most adolescents say that they communicate well with parents on all issues, including their most pressing problems and concerns. Further, most adolescents share their parents' values and attitudes toward moral and political issues. They frequently turn to their parents for guidance, particularly about their most important academic, career, and personal choices. (Damon, 1983, p. 265)

Additionally, there is overlap between parental and peer values because the adolescent's friends are likely to have the same background. Parental influence is more important than peer influence when parents express affection, interest, understanding, and a willingness to be helpful (Mussen, 1979). Support from parents is positively associated with adolescents' beliefs about locus of control (internal versus external) (Scheck, Emerick, and El-Assal, 1973). It is also positively associated with the ability of the adolescent to experience empathy (Adams et al., 1982).

Developmental Considerations

During adolescence, the nature of the relationship between parents and children changes. The relationship shifts from one that is primarily hierarchical to one that is more symmetrical. William Damon (1983), based on his review of the literature on adolescent relationships, suggests that adolescents transfer skills that they have learned in peer relations to this new relationship with their parents. This shift to a symmetrical relationship between parents and adolescent children can create some initial adjustment difficulties. From an attachment perspective, as suggested in the preceding chapter, there is a transformation in the parent-adolescent relationship: adolescents are motivated to become less emotionally dependent on their parents.

PARENTING STRATEGIES

Parenting strategies influence the nature of the parent-adolescent relationship. For example, Patricia Noller (1994) reports on the influence of physical punishment and other parenting strategies on adolescent functioning:

- Physical punishment of adolescents promotes external locus of control, low self-confidence, social isolation, and covert resentment or rebellion.
- Neglectful and inconsistent discipline seems to increase the likelihood of delinquent behavior.
- Autocratic parenting tends to make adolescents more dependent and less self-confident.

• Severe and inconsistent discipline combined with an unhappy relationship between parents increases the likelihood that an adolescent child will engage in rebellious behavior.

After reviewing research in this area, Noller (1994) concluded, "Once again it seems clear that the balance between support and control is the crucial issue in parenting adolescents. High support and low to moderate control seem to provide the ideal environment for healthy adolescents" (p. 47).

Parenting Styles

Diana Baumrind (1978) identified three parenting styles that have been investigated extensively: *authoritarian, permissive,* and *authoritative or democratic.*

1. *Authoritarian Parenting Style.* A high value is place on obedience, so parents rely on strategies that are punitive to promote subordination. These parents are detached, controlling, and demanding. Relative to others, these children are more likely to be discontented, withdrawn, and distrustful.
2. *Permissive Parenting Style.* Parents rely on strategies that are noncontrolling and nondemanding. Compared to others, these children are less self-reliant, explorative, and self-controlled.
3. *Authoritative or Democratic Parenting Style.* Baumrind described this as a unique combination of high control and positive encouragement of autonomy and independence. Parents seem to value self-will of their children and try to help their children make rational choices. Compared to others, these children are more self-reliant, self-controlled, and explorative.

In adolescence, authoritative or democratic parenting is associated with the greatest social competence. This parenting style is also positively associated with identity-achievement formation.

A clinician should evaluate parental discipline style (see Table 6.1). Behavioral characteristics of the adolescent may be an efficient form of assessment (e.g., if the adolescent acts aggressively toward the therapist, the parents may use either dictatorial or indifferent styles of parenting), which can be used to develop interventions.

TABLE 6.1. Impact of Parent Discipline Style

Parent's Discipline Style	Impact on Adolescent
Overprotective or indulgent	Polite, neat, and dependent
Dictatorial and antagonistic	Withdrawn, neurotic, and antagonistic
Democratic and cooperative	Highly sociable and independent
Indifferent and detached	Noncompliant and aggressive

Source: Based on Becker (1964).

Ironically, parental intentions may be unwittingly contra-dicted by the chosen discipline style. For example, Erin's parents monitored her behavior excessively because they were afraid "she's going to get into more trouble. If she'd behave responsibly, we'd cut her some slack." Their "monitoring" evolved into a dictatorial and anta-gonistic parenting style, so Erin withdrew from the family, made sarcastic comments to her parents, and violated family rules.

From a family systems perspective, parenting style can account for different behavior in children from the same family; this often results in one child being scapegoated or identified as the problem. For a variety of reasons, some accidental, some deliberate, some conscious, some unconscious, parents may discipline their children differently. It is important for the clinician to help families recognize these differences in order to help parents change their discipline style.

SOLUTION-FOCUSED PARENTING

From the previous discussion on parenting styles, it seems clear that one would want to promote an authoritative or democratic parenting style and that one would want to foster attachment relationships between adolescents and their parents by cultivating a secure family base. Toni Schindler Zimmerman and her colleagues (1996) at Colorado State University have developed an innovative approach to teaching parenting skills that is based on principles of solution-focused therapy. They have tested it with families of adolescents, and results suggest that it has a positive influence. This section will review the key aspects of a solution-focused approach to therapy, review the Zimmerman curriculum, and discuss clinical implications for family therapy with adolescents.

Principles of Solution-Focused Therapy

Solution-focused therapy is influenced by the belief that clients have strengths and resources that should be utilized in therapy. This approach is based on the following assumptions (de Shazer et al., 1986; de Shazer and Molnar, 1984; O'Hanlon and Weiner-Davis, 1989):

- Most complaints develop in the context of human interaction.
- Any problem can be interpreted in a variety of ways.
- Only small change is necessary.
- Change in one part of the system leads to change in the system as a whole.
- Clients have resources and strengths to resolve their complaints.
- Change is constant.
- The therapist should identify and amplify change.
- It is usually unnecessary to know a great deal about the complaint in order to resolve it.
- It is not necessary to know the cause or function of a complaint to resolve it.
- Clients define the goals of therapy.
- Rapid change or resolution of problems is possible.
- There is no one "right" way to view things; different views may be just as valid and may fit the facts just as well.
- Therapy should focus on what is possible and changeable, rather than what is impossible and intractable.

Several useful interventions have been developed that incorporate a solution-focused approach to therapy: *the formula first session task, search for exceptions, the miracle question, normalizing,* and *presuppositional questioning.* The following discussion of these interventions are based on the work of de Shazer and colleagues (de Shazer et al., 1986; de Shazer and Molnar, 1984) and O'Hanlon and Weiner-Davis (1989).

The Formula First Session Task

The goal of the formula first session task is to help clients see problems as changeable, rather than to focus on perceived stability of problematic patterns. Intervention: "Between now and the next time we meet, observe aspects of your life/relationship that you want to continue" (O'Hanlon and Weiner-Davis, 1989, p. 23). This intervention suggests that change is expected.

Search for Exceptions

As in the first task, the goal of the search for exceptions intervention is to help the client see that problems are not fixed and that, in fact, there are already times when the problem does not exist. Therapists either directly ask clients to tell them about times when they have not experienced the problem or follow up on examples provided by clients. After exceptions have been identified, therapists ask a variety of follow-up questions to reinforce the idea that the client has already identified some solutions. Examples include, "How do you get that to happen? How does it make your day go differently?"

The Miracle Question

If clients are unable to identify exceptions, therapists ask clients to pretend that a miracle had occurred and the problem had disappeared. Once clients have been able to fulfill this request, therapists ask a variety of follow-up questions that are intended to identify different behaviors that could be used to solve the problem.

Normalizing

Normalizing is a very helpful intervention for families that include adolescents. Using material from various chapters in this book, parents can learn to recognize aspects of adolescent development that are fairly typical so that they can relax or refrain from overreacting to a problem.

Presuppositional Questioning

Presuppositional questioning is used to suggest that change is inevitable. These are likened to "leading" questions used by attorneys. Reflection upon these questions helps clients to consider their situations from new perspectives.

Themes in Solution-Focused Parenting

Toni Zimmerman and colleagues (1996) developed a six-week solution-focused parenting group for parents of adolescents that seemed to improve parenting skills and family functioning. The details of their program are available from Dr. Zimmerman.[4] Themes from their program that can be incorporated into family therapy will be reviewed. (The following material is based on Zimmerman et al., 1996.)

Session 1: Family Strengths and Inevitability of Change

The transition from childhood to adolescence is normalized as inevitable and parents are introduced to the assumptions of solution-focused parenting, which are consistent with those briefly reviewed earlier in this section. As parents identify adolescent problem behavior, facilitators identify family strengths that could be used to address them.

Session 2: Pebbles in the Pond Versus Niagara Falls (Small Changes)

Parents are asked to identify positive behaviors engaged in by their adolescent children. Facilitators suggest to participants that these positive behaviors—identified as small changes—could be used as a foundation for solving larger problems. Facilitators also suggest to parents that their feedback contributes to the maintenance of adolescent behavior and encourages the parents to focus on these newly identified positive behaviors. Parents are asked to choose one small goal and to keep a record of behaviors and activities that support this small goal.

Session 3: Building Upon What Works

Facilitators follow up on the goals set during the previous session. Parents are encouraged to continue to build on successes.

Facilitators also discuss interactional cycles and suggest to parents that these cycles could be interrupted at any point during the cycle. Parents are asked to think about solution-focused ways to interrupt the cycle. Facilitators also suggest to parents that "backsliding" is normal and encourage them to remain optimistic about building on small changes.

Session 4: If It Doesn't Work, Do Something Different

As in the previous week, facilitators inquire about positive behaviors and encourage parents to continue to use their supportive strategies. If parents are unable to identify successful strategies, facilitators engage them in brainstorming alternative strategies. These parents are encouraged to "do something different" in their parenting.

Session 5: Keep Change Happening
(Being Open to Many Solutions)

Facilitators continue to explore exceptions to family problems and to amplify positive strategies. A family of origin perspective is also introduced to normalize parenting strategies. Participants are asked to identify parenting strategies that they have incorporated, consciously or unconsciously, from their own parents. Participants are asked to evaluate the utility of these strategies and to develop alternative behaviors in order to have a more diverse repertoire of parenting responses to a variety of problems.

Session 6: Celebrating Change

Facilitators congratulate participants for changes that have been experienced and encourage them to identify specific parenting strategies that reinforce change. Assumptions of solution-focused parenting are also reviewed for participants.

Compared to nonparticipants, results suggest that parents who participate in this program demonstrate improvement on the following dimensions of parenting: building rapport, communication, and setting limits. Each of these dimensions are associated with attachment, so it seems reasonable to expect that encouraging parents to adopt solution-focused parenting skills will foster attachment behavior and bonds in families.

SUMMARY

Aspects of the parent-adolescent relationship that influence attachment and family functioning have been reviewed. Several assessment devices to help measure family relationships were identified and an approach to parenting that incorporates principles of solution-focused therapy was discussed. It was suggested that this solution-focused parenting would facilitate attachment relationships.

Chapter 7

Peer Relationships

The developmental-systemic model recognizes that peers make important contributions to adolescent development. Parents often express concern about peer influence: they seem inclined to blame their adolescent's friends if the child engages in some kind of delinquent behavior. Since this is a common concern, this chapter begins by looking at peer influence. It then turns to two other important aspects of peer relationships: friendship relationships and peer rejection.

PEER INFLUENCE

Peer Orientation

Generally, adolescent males and females report similar perceptions of peer pressure, but males are more likely to submit to peer influence (Brown, Clasen, and Eicher, 1986). Conger (1971), after completing a review of the literature on peer influence, concluded that peer influence will supersede parent influence when (a) there is a strong, homogeneous group that has attitudes and behaviors that are very different from those of parents; (b) there is not a rewarding parent-child relationship; (c) parental values are uninformed, inconsistent, unrealistic, maladaptive, or hypocritical; and (d) the adolescent lacks self-confidence or independence training to resist peer influence.

Conger (1971) continues: "the peer-oriented child is more a product of parental disregard than of the attractiveness of the peer group . . . he turns to his agemate less by choice than by default. The vacuum left by the withdrawal of parents and adults from the lives of children is filled with . . . the substitute of an age-segregated peer group" (pp. 1128-1129). As a result, parental concern about peer pressure should be examined in therapy as a parent-adolescent problem. Remember Erin and Chris?[1] Erin's parents were justifiably concerned that she was sneaking out at night to drive around with her friends. It was fortunate that Erin was not injured when she and her friends drove around getting high. Chris' sexual behavior was a problem for his mother because it contradicted her personal values and put him at risk for HIV/AIDS; he was also putting his dating partners at risk for pregnancy and sexually transmitted disease.

Sources of Influence

The level of peer and parent influence seems to be affected by topic. Peer influence is strongest for matters of taste in music, fashion, language, and peer interaction. Parent influence, on the other hand, seems to have a stronger influence on issues of moral and social values, and views of the world. This information can be used to reassure parents by normalizing peer influence.

The W family, that included a fourteen-year-old girl named Emily, initiated therapy because the parents were concerned about the influence of Emily's friend, Amanda. When Emily received two failing grades on her midterm report card, her parents attributed the academic problems to Amanda. Emily and Amanda had recently adopted a "Goth" style of dress. Emily's parents concluded that the change in clothing was responsible for a change in their daughter's attitude about school, so they told Emily that she would no longer be allowed to dress in the Goth style. Her parents also concluded that these changes were ultimately the responsibility of Amanda, whom they described as "a bad influence on Emily."

Amanda, who had also received poor grades, was punished in a similar manner by her mother, who was a single parent, so the two girls decided to run away from home. The girls initially spent one night with their friend June.[2] Emily's parents contacted the parents of Emily's friends when they discovered that she had run away, but June's parents were unaware that Emily and Amanda were at their home. June's parents promised to contact the Ws if they came in contact with Emily. When June's mother discovered Emily and Amanda asleep the next morning, she called the Ws.

The Ws were visibly upset when they entered the office. Emily avoided eye contact. After telling me about the recent events, Mr. W expressed concern: "I'm afraid we're losing our girl. I don't know who this stubborn, petulant person is that has taken over my daughter's body, but she's driving me crazy!"

I was concerned that the Ws, who were legitimately concerned about their daughter's welfare, may have overreacted to the initial problem, which was poor grades. "It seems to me that we have two sets of problems here, although it might seem to you that you've got just one. First, we need to address Emily's running away for safety reasons. It also seems as if we need to address the problem that started the ball rolling on this series of events: responding to poor grades. Which one would you like to talk about first?"

Mr. W responded gruffly, "We don't have two problems. We have one problem: Emily has become more and more disobedient and it's that Amanda's fault. She's the one who has been a bad influence on our daughter and I'm not going to sit around and let her screw up my daughter's life!"

The words hung in the air as I paused to collect my thoughts. Emily had clearly made a bad decision and the family needed to provide a logical consequence for running away from home. I was concerned that blaming Amanda would minimize Emily's responsibility, and, if we wanted to help her make better decisions in the future, it seemed to me that we should focus on her part in the process. "Emily, could you tell me what happened when you decided to run away from home?"

"Not much to tell. We were mad at our parents so we decided to spend the night at June's. No big deal."

Mr. W exploded. "What do you mean no big deal? Do you have any idea how upset your mother and I were? No big deal? We called the police. We called all of your friends. Do you know how stupid I felt calling other parents and asking them if they'd seen my daughter?" Emily cringed but said nothing.

This time the words seemed to echo around the room during a long pause. I tried again, directing my words toward Mr. W. "I'm concerned that if we only focus on Amanda, Emily will lose the opportunity to take responsibility for her own decision." I looked at Mr. W who made no response. I turned to Emily. "OK. So, Emily, you and Amanda were mad at your parents so you decided to run away. What were you mad about?"

"Amanda's mom told her that we couldn't be friends and my folks said that I couldn't hang out with Amanda anymore. They also started yelling at me about the way I dressed, as if that affected my grades."

I sensed that Mr. W was becoming more agitated. "Whose idea was it to spend the night at June's?"

"I don't know. We were both talking about how mad we were at our parents and I guess I said something like, 'I can't stand to be in this house' and then I called June to see if she would let me spend the night."

"I'd like to clarify two points. First of all, you said that you called June to see if she would let you spend the night. So did you think that what you were doing was running away from home or spending the night with a friend?"

"I thought I was spending the night with a friend," she replied.

"Your parents were upset. They were frightened because they didn't know where you were. They called the police because they thought you'd run away from home. Did you think about that? Why didn't you tell them you were going to spend the night at June's?"

"How could I tell them? I was grounded so they wouldn't let me spend the night at June's, but I was so mad that I had to get out of the house. I was upset. I guess that I didn't think about them."

"I want to clarify another point. Your parents have said that Amanda is a bad influence. They see your running away as an example of her influence. How much did Amanda influence your decision to leave the house?"

Emily's tone became more firm. "That's just it. First of all, like I said, I didn't run away. I spent the night at a friend's house. Second of all, Amanda didn't make me do anything. I was mad at my folks so I decided to go to June's. Amanda didn't make me do anything. It was my decision."

"Now, are you sure you want to admit to that? Wouldn't it be easier for you to blame Amanda?"

"It wasn't Amanda's fault. I'm not some silly little girl whose friends can brainwash her or push her around. I was mad so I left the house. That was wrong. I shouldn't have left without telling Mom and Dad, but I don't think they were being fair. Go ahead and ground me or something, but don't tell me who to have as a friend."

This case demonstrates the complexities associated with parenting an adolescent. It also demonstrates the need for parents to develop logical consequences rather than arbitrary ones. Rather than investigate factors associated with the poor grades, the Ws inferred that Emily's poor grades were the result of her clothes and her friends. They responded by telling Emily that she would have to change her clothing style and her friends. This decision set in motion Emily's decision to leave the house. In the remainder of this chapter, additional aspects of peer relationships are discussed.

FRIENDS

In Chapter 5, it was noted that friends are a source of attachment in adolescence. Friends help adolescents by providing them with "a sense of belonging that enhances their sense of well-being. Having a companion for activities makes adolescents' lives more enjoyable. In these and other ways, a close friend enhances adolescents' well-being" (Berndt, 1996, p. 77). There are direct benefits to adolescents who have supportive friends. For example, recall the research of Susan Harter on self-esteem (Chapter 4). Her research suggests that physical attractiveness has a stronger influence on self-esteem for adolescents who lack friends. Steven R. Asher (1990) has studied adolescent relationships extensively. He writes, "Friends are important sources of companionship and recreation, share advice and valued possessions, serve as trusted confidants and critics, act as loyal allies, and provide stability in times of stress and transition" (p. 3).

After reviewing research on adolescent friendships, Thomas J. Berndt (1996) concluded that supportive friendships have four qualities. First, friends provide *informational support* or advice about problems. Second, friends provide *instrumental support* by providing help on projects such as homework or other tasks. Third, friends provide *companionship support* by participating in joint activities. Fourth, friends provide *esteem support* by providing encouragement, congratulations, and other forms of emotional support. Each of these activities promotes intimacy.

PEER REJECTION

Some adolescents lack supportive friendships and seem to be actively rejected by their peers. This rejection is associated with negative consequences. In this section, factors associated with peer rejection are identified and the consequences of peer rejection are discussed.

Consequences of Peer Rejection

John D. Coie (1990), after reviewing research in this area, identified consequences of peer rejection:

1. Peer rejection increases stress and loneliness. Peers are more likely to ignore or behave aggressively toward the rejected adolescent.
2. Peer-rejected adolescents have fewer coping skills. "Because of their relative isolation from peers as they move into adolescence, rejected children are likely to be deprived of opportunities to develop social competencies that might enable them to cope effectively" (Coie, 1990, p. 370).
3. Rejected adolescents have lower self-esteem. (The significance of self-esteem was discussed at length in Chapter 4.)
4. Peer rejection seems to promote problems at school. Adolescents who experience peer rejection are more likely to skip school, do poorly in their work, and are more likely to drop out of school. Teachers report having more difficulty disciplining peer-rejected adolescents.

Factors Associated with Peer Rejection

It seems clear that peer rejection is a significant problem for some adolescents, and that it might help therapists create interventions if the factors that seem to influence it are understood. This section identifies factors that seem to promote initial rejection by peers. The following section discusses factors that seem to maintain peer rejection. Physical characteristics are often a source for peer teasing, but they are not typically the main reason children are rejected by their peers. Children who are initially rejected by their peers seem to be either aggressive and disruptive or socially withdrawn (Coie, 1990).

The development of aggressive or withdrawn characteristics are influenced by parent relationships such as *attachment* and *reinforcement history* (Coie, 1990). The extent to which these characteristics are amplified by peers and contribute to peer rejection seems to be associated with *situation-specific social skills* (Coie, 1990).

Attachment

Recall from the discussion on attachment in Chapter 5 that attachment has three interdependent dimensions: attachment behavior, attachment behavioral system, and attachment bond (Cassidy, 1999). Coie addresses the attachment bond: "The degree to which parent and child have a strong attachment bond is predictive of the extent to which the child can experience intimacy in future relationships. Rubin and his colleagues take this premise further and speculate that the type of attachment bond will be predictive of the type of peer relationship" (1990, p. 391).

In addition to attachment bond, attachment behaviors with caregivers are likely to be used in some modified form with peers. This suggests that behaviors associated with insecure attachment, especially avoidant (children) or dismissing (adolescents and adults) attachment, might promote peer rejection. R. Rogers Kobak and Amy Sceery (1988) examined attachment in later adolescence using the Adult Attachment Interview (details about the AAI are provided in Chapter 5). Participants identified as demonstrating a dismissive adult attachment style were more likely to be rated by peers as hostile (Kobak and Sceery, 1988); hostility is a trait that has been associated with peer rejection. Participants who demonstrated a dismissive attachment style also reported more loneliness and low levels of social support from their families. These factors are also associated with peer rejection.

This suggests that if an adolescent is experiencing problems with peers, attachment relationships should be assessed. If there are problems associated with attachment, they should be addressed at some level in therapy with the family.

Reinforcement History

Peer rejection also seems to be influenced by social skills that are usually learned from parents, who are role models and sources of reinforcement. Coie (1990) elaborates: "Through mechanisms of modeling, coaching, and operant conditioning, parents influence the acquisition of social behaviors and social skills that their children then display in peer social encounters" (p. 392). In contrast to peer rejection associated with attachment, in these cases we might want to emphasize learning and practicing social skills. Social skill training is often done as part of a psychoeducational program developed for adolescents. It may be more relevant, though, to address these in family therapy so that parents can serve as role models and be encouraged to reinforce these behaviors in their adolescent children.

Situation-Specific Social Skills

Some adolescents experience peer rejection because they lack appropriate social skills that are required for specific situations. Some children are able to manage some situations but seem to struggle managing others. This is idiosyncratic to the child. In these cases, the therapist should identify specific situations in which the adolescent struggles and address social skills related to it. This was exemplified in a case that was discussed in the chapter on identity (Chapter 3). Troy was at risk for being rejected by his peers because he taunted them about grades. I consulted with Troy only briefly as we looked at specific ways he could respond differently to his peers about grades.

Factors Associated with Continued Peer Rejection

Despite their negative experiences with peers, rejected children and adolescents do not seem to change their behavior. In order to develop clinical interventions, one should examine reasons why peer rejection persists. In addition to identifying consequences of peer rejection and factors associated with it, John Coie (1990) also discovered four factors associated with continued peer rejection: *lack of knowledge about obtaining skills, motivation, limited reinforcement for change,* and *self-fulfilling prophecy.* The following discussion is based on his review.

Lack of Knowledge About Obtaining Skills

As previously noted, adolescents who are rejected by their peers lack social skills. They also seem to be unaware of resources that might help them learn these skills. This suggests that assessment of social skills should be a routine part of assessment of adolescents. In cases where the client seems to lack social skills, some component in therapy that helps facilitate acquisition of social skills should be included. Interventions designed to improve social skills are described later in this chapter.

Motivation

Rejected adolescents may not recognize that they are experiencing atypical relationships, so they may not be motivated to change. This reinforces the need for therapists to conduct an assessment of friendships and school relations with all of their adolescent clients.

Limited Reinforcement for Change

Once adolescents have been rejected by their peers, it is often difficult to change the perceptions of peers: "Once a child is categorized as disliked, positive acts by that child are more likely to be attributed to external causes. . . . Thus, rejected children who attempt to alter their negative impact on peers have an uphill climb ahead of them and may be inclined to give up and revert to old solutions" (Coie, 1990, p. 384). This suggests that any attempts to improve social skills should include encouragement to be persistent.

Self-Fulfilling Prophecy

As just noted, peers are unlikely to notice change in the behavior of a rejected adolescent. In some cases, the rejected adolescent serves the function of group scapegoat, which will make the task of obtaining peer acceptance even more difficult. In these cases, one might want to normalize frustrations when efforts are ignored or even fail, so that the adolescent is encouraged to be persistent.

ASSESSMENT OF PEER REJECTION

In the previous section, it was noted that assessment of social skills should be a routine part of treatment with adolescents. Before looking at interventions, methods of assessment are discussed. Informally, one would want to ask about adolescents' friendships as well as peer relations at school. There are also formal assessment instruments that might be helpful. One might want to assess peer attachment since it is associated with peer rejection. The Inventory of Parent and Peer Attachment (IPPA) was discussed in Chapter 5 (Armsden and Greenberg, 1987). The IPPA is a self-report measure of attachment for adolescents, which includes a twenty-five-item scale that measures attachment to close friends.

It might also be helpful to assess feelings of loneliness as well as perception of social support. Steven R. Asher, who is one of the leading researchers on peer relationships, has developed the Children's Loneliness Scale (CLS), which is a self-report measure that assesses perception of loneliness (Asher and Wheeler, 1985). The scale is developmentally appropriate for adolescents. It includes twenty-four questions, but eight of them are "filler" items that are included to help children feel more comfortable completing the instrument. Each question is based on a five-point scale. The CLS demonstrates excellent reliability (both consistency and test-retest stability) and validity.[3]

The Social Support Appraisals Scale (SSA) developed by Alan Vaux and his colleagues (Vaux et al., 1986) is another helpful assessment measure. It includes twenty-three questions that are designed to assess perception of affection and support from family and friends. The scale is developmentally appropriate, reliable, and clinically valid.[4]

CLINICAL INTERVENTION FOR PEER REJECTION

Kenneth W. Merrell and Gretchen A. Gimpel, in their book *Social Skills of Children and Adolescents* (1998), contend that social skills are learned through observation, modeling, rehearsal, and receiving feedback. They also suggest that effective social skills require initiating conversation and responding to conversation in ways that are expected and appropriate.

Interventions designed to help rejected adolescents have focused on helping the client learn social skills. This may occur in a traditional psychoeducational format or may be included as a part of family therapy with adolescents. In this section, aspects for intervention that could be used in both formats are reviewed. Specific social skills are reviewed, and distinct aspects associated with adolescents who are aggressive versus those who are socially withdrawn (since these are the two groups most likely to experience peer rejection) are discussed.

Social Skills Categories

From a solution-focused perspective, it may be helpful to identify types of social skills that an adolescent seems to have already learned and used. When working with rejected adolescents or others who seem to struggle in interpersonal relationships, it may be helpful to identify specific areas in which they have difficulty. To help identify strengths and areas for growth, it may be helpful to distinguish between categories of social skills. Four categories of social skills seem to be important for adolescents who have been rejected by their peers: *peer relationship skills, self-management skills, academic skills,* and *assertion skills.*

Peer Relationship Skills

Rejected adolescents may have difficulty interacting with their peers in ways that are positive. The therapist should seek to promote skills in which the adolescent learns to compliment and praise peers, learns to ask for assistance and initiate activities, and is sensitive to the feelings of others (Merrell and Gimpel, 1998). In therapy, family members could practice these activities with one another. In addition to practicing a skill, these behaviors may improve family dynamics.

Self-Management Skills

Adolescents who are rejected due to aggressive behavior may need to focus on self-management skills such as controlling their temper, following rules, accepting compromises, and responding to critical feedback. One might want to focus in particular on helping adolescent clients remain calm when faced with problems, especially if they are teased by their peers (Merrell and Gimpel, 1998). For socially withdrawn adolescents, the therapist should help them respond to teasing with a sense of humor rather than with isolation.

Academic Skills

Because the classroom is a social environment, academic skills influence peer relations in several ways. For example, peers often tease others who are not prepared for class or laugh when someone makes a mistake. In these situations, an aggressive response or an isolating response may make the situation worse. This suggests that the therapist should inquire about the following academic skills: ability to complete tasks independently and on time, listen to and complete instructions, use free time appropriately, ask for assistance, and ignore peer distractions (Merrell and Gimpel, 1998). Aggressive adolescents may experience more difficulty responding to peer distractions and using free time appropriately. Socially withdrawn adolescents may struggle to ask for help.

Assertion Skills

Both aggressive and socially withdrawn adolescents may struggle to be appropriately assertive. These skills include initiating conversations, acknowledging compliments, inviting peers to engage in activities, saying and doing nice things for others, initiating contact with new people, and expressing hurt feelings appropriately (Merrell and Gimpel, 1998). Aggressive adolescents may initiate contact with peers in ways that are interpreted by others as invasive, so they should be helped to soften the ways in which they approach others. On the other hand, socially withdrawn adolescents may need coaching just to attempt to make contact. This could be particularly intimidating to withdrawn adolescents who are not accustomed to interacting with others.

Aggressive Adolescents

Adolescents who seem to be aggressive might benefit from an improvement in all of the social skill categories. Merrell and Gimpel (1998) recommend a cognitive problem-solving approach to teaching social skills to those identified as aggressive. They identify five characteristics associated with this type of approach that can be easily incorporated into family therapy sessions (Merrell and Gimpel, 1998):

1. Focus on thought processes rather than behavior.
2. Provide a step-by-step approach to dealing with particular situations.
3. Incorporate structured tasks as a way to teach skills.
4. Therapist should be an active participant in the process.
5. Therapist provides modeling and feedback. Experiential activities such as role plays are used to practice skills.

Socially Withdrawn Adolescents

For socially withdrawn adolescents one might want to focus on peer relationship, self-management, and assertion skills because these children usually demonstrate academic and compliance skills. Merrell and Gimpel (1998) make two specific suggestions for improving social skills of adolescents who are socially withdrawn:

1. Assess reasons for social withdrawal. Some children may have social skills but may have difficulty using them with their peers.
2. Ensure that participants have the opportunity to practice newly acquired skills in "real-life" situations.

In addition to these two suggestions, one might also want to address feelings, especially fears that adolescents have about interacting with peers. Feelings associated with rejection are particularly strong for socially withdrawn adolescents who have been rejected by their peers. Experiential techniques discussed in Chapter 2 might be helpful in these situations.

SUMMARY

Parents are often concerned about peer pressure but there are other aspects of peer relationships that should be assessed during therapy with adolescents. Most of this chapter was spent discussing peer rejection because it is associated with serious negative consequences for adolescent development.

SECTION III:
ADOLESCENT RISK TAKING

Chapter 8

Sexuality

Parents are often, at best, mildly anxious about the emerging sexuality of their children. In most cases, adolescent sexual attitudes and behaviors are serious matters in families. A colleague recently related the story of a couple whose seventeen-year-old daughter's sexual behavior created conflict between the parents. The daughter confided in her mother that she had recently started engaging in sexual intercourse with her long-time boyfriend. The mother related this information to her husband.

Conflict occurred between the couple because they disagreed about how to respond to their daughter's disclosure. The mother, noting that she and her husband had engaged in intercourse prior to marriage, advocated for a pragmatic approach. She suggested that they should counsel their daughter to "take precautions" if the girl was going to be sexually active. The father, on the other hand, insisted that they should forbid their daughter to see the boyfriend. The parents were clearly concerned about their daughter because engaging in sexual intercourse put the young woman at risk for pregnancy and HIV/AIDS. Premarital sexual intercourse also violated deeply held religious convictions of the parents. They consulted with my colleague because they reported that this disagreement was creating marital conflict.

The therapist consulted only briefly with the family. He suggested to the couple that their goals were similar in that they both wanted to protect their daughter. He further recommended that they should think carefully about forbidding the daughter to see the boyfriend because that approach might make the situation worse by putting the daughter in the position of defending the young man, which could increase her loyalty to him. The therapist further recommended to the couple that they share their concerns honestly with their daughter and even relate to her that they had engaged in premarital sexual intercourse.

The father was initially reluctant because he feared that if his daughter knew the truth, she would use that information to justify her own behavior. This is fairly common: parents are often reluctant to discuss their behavior as youth for fear that their children will "use this as ammunition." In fact, sharing this information—a type of *leveling* with children—seems to increase parent credibility. Rather than losing respect or using the information against their parents, adolescents seem to feel a sense of validation that their parents are willing to talk to them rather than lecture them. (The importance of this is discussed later in the chapter when results from focus groups with adolescents are reviewed.)

The therapist also suggested to the couple that they talk to the boyfriend as well. This seemed to be particularly important because young women are often "gatekeepers" for sexual expression in dating relationships. Discussing the sexual relationship with the young man put him in a position of being responsible sexually.

This chapter reviews research on adolescent sexual attitudes and behaviors, and information that can be used clinically to normalize adolescent sexual experience. This chapter also discusses recommendations for intervention, based on focus groups about adolescent sexuality conducted with parents and adolescents (Werner-Wilson and Coughlin-Smith, 1997).

As previously noted, parents should be concerned about the sexual behavior of their adolescent children because contemporary adolescents are faced with potentially severe consequences for engaging in risky sexual behaviors. Research on adolescent sexuality has identified the following long-term outcomes associated with teen pregnancy and teen parenthood:

- Teen parents are ill prepared for parenting (Barret and Robinson, 1982; Cannon-Bonaventure and Kahn, 1979; De Lissovoy, 1973).
- Teen marriages are more likely to end in divorce (De Lissovoy, 1973; Furstenberg, 1976).

• Teen mothers are especially handicapped due to limited education and employment opportunities (Furstenberg, Levine, and
Brooks-Gunn, 1990).

Today, sexual experimentation is associated with severe health
risks including sexually transmitted diseases, especially the risk of
contracting the HIV/AIDS virus. Parents are keenly aware of these
consequences and, according to our focus groups, they report a
great deal of anxiety about these threats (Werner-Wilson and
Coughlin-Smith, 1997). Despite these concerns, research suggests
that many parents are reluctant to talk to their adolescent children
about sexuality. Furthermore, the way parents approach talking
about sex seems to undermine the conversation. This research is
discussed in more detail as factors that influence adolescent sexuality are reviewed and clinical implications are discussed.

Adolescent sexual attitudes and behavior are influenced by four
factors that are relevant to family therapy with adolescents: *media,
individual psychosocial factors, dating dynamics,* and *family relationships.*

MEDIA INFLUENCES

Adolescents are active consumers of messages broadcast on radio
and television, printed in magazines, distributed on the Internet, and
produced in video games. How do these influences compete with
parental guidance? Popular media may replace more worthwhile activities and passively reinforce gender and ethnic stereotypes (Gerber
et al., 1986; R. J. Wilson, 1990). For example, I conducted a content
analysis of *Rolling Stone* magazine, a periodical popular with adolescents, which examined gender and ethnic themes in issues published in
the years 1968 and 1988. Women and people from traditionally under-
represented groups were rarely the source of stories; when they were
featured, they were depicted unflatteringly.

Television seems to be the more powerful and insidious medium,
so its influence is the focus of the remainder of this section. On
average, children will witness 8,000 murders and 100,000 acts of
violence on television *before* they enter middle school (Huston et al.,
1992). Viewing violence in sexual contexts is associated with acceptance of rape and other forms of violence (Huston et al., 1992).

Victor C. Strasburger is a pediatrician and adolescent medicine specialist who has written a book titled *Adolescents and the Media: Medical and Psychological Impact* (Strasburger, 1995). Bradley S. Greenberg and colleagues (Greenberg, Brown, and Buerkel-Roth-fuss, 1993) have edited another book on the topic titled *Media, Sex, and the Adolescent*. Strasburger concludes that television and other media are the leading source of sex education in the United States because there is no widespread, effective sex education program. Parents, then friends, then media, are typically considered to be the most significant influences on adolescent attitudes and behaviors. After reviewing research in this area, both books report that sexual content is becoming increasingly graphic and common on television. Also, research suggests that increased viewing of television influences sexual attitudes and behaviors: adolescents who watch more television are more likely to experiment sexually and report that they have had intercourse.

Television viewing can change emotions, so people may use television to manipulate their feelings. For example, a bored adolescent may watch MTV, which bombards the viewer with images, for stimulation. Watching television can also help viewers learn to identify emotions (Zillmann, 1982). Unfortunately, it is likely that the representations will be inaccurate so adolescents may develop a skewed understanding of complex emotional processes. Research suggests that adolescents watch television for two primary reasons (Huston et al., 1992):

1. *Default hypothesis:* adolescents watch television because they have nothing better to do.
2. *Displacement hypothesis:* adolescents watch television as a substitute for other activities.

Media Influence: Clinical Implications

Clinicians should recognize the power of the media and be aware of its messages. Moreover, therapists should watch television shows that are produced for adolescent audiences in order to develop an understanding of the ever-changing adolescent culture. How do these programs address sexuality, violence, independence, family relationships, group memberships? The television shows can be starting points for conversation in therapy.

Although most parents express concern about the influence of the media, few of them seem to actually take time to watch television, listen to music, or browse the Internet with their children. I often assign a homework task to encourage parent-adolescent interaction about media messages. I ask parents to spend time participating in media-related activities with their children. This task seems to address both the default and displacement hypotheses because it provides alternative activities (e.g., parent-adolescent interaction) to isolated media consumption. As a result of this assignment, adolescents seem to become more aware of messages in the media, which, in turn, often prompts them to discontinue interacting with some media on their own.

Stephanie, a single parent, and her only son, David, reported that a constant source of conflict was the music that David enjoyed. Stephanie seemed to complain that the music was either "too loud" or, overhearing a lyric, "offensive." David typically ignored his mother or told her that she was "overreacting" because "it's just a song." I asked her to begin listening to music with him, but I encouraged her to try to listen without criticizing it. Instead, I prompted her to ask David about the music, and if she found something offensive, to explain her reasons to David and ask his opinion about the particular song. Initially, David continued to tell Stephanie that she was overreacting, but the more she joined him in listening to music, the less he seemed to play songs that Stephanie found offensive.

In another case, Internet browsing became a concern. The F family initiated therapy because Steve, a fourteen-year-old, was having academic difficulties. Ann, who was a single mother, and Mitch, Steve's younger brother, attended sessions with Steve. Steve had been a solid B student in his first year of middle school but he failed three classes during the initial term of his second year. Ann told me that she was concerned about the amount of time that Steve spent browsing the Internet and participating in chat rooms. She indicated that she had found him looking at sexually explicit material on several occasions. In each case, Steve claimed that he was working on a term paper but the search engine had directed him to the particular site.

I asked where the computer was located in the house and was told that Steve had moved it to his room during the summer because he was the primary user and he said that he could not concentrate when he tried to use it in the family room. I asked about amount of usage. Ann reported, "He's on the computer all the time. I can sometimes hear him typing past midnight." Steve also seemed to have difficulty waking up for school.

Given this information, we talked about options. I started by suggesting that Steve's interest in the Internet was a sign of curiosity and a desire to learn. "Isn't it ironic, though, that Steve's interest in learning might be interfering with school where learning is a primary goal?" I asked. "Should we look for ways that Steve could use the Internet to help him with school and to satisfy his curiosity that don't interfere with school?" Ann and Steve identified four options: (1) move the computer out of Steve's room; (2) limit the amount of time that Steve spent on the computer; (3) discontinue Internet access; or (4) sell the computer.

Steve objected to each option, claiming that moving the computer out of his room or restricting his usage would interfere with his ability to complete schoolwork. I suspected that Steve had not been accidentally directed to Internet sites that featured sexually explicit material, but I saw no need to confront him about his interest in this kind of material. I have found that moving a computer with Internet access to a public space in the home seems to reduce the frequency of these "accidents," so I asked if there were alternatives to either the family room or Steve's bedroom. "Is there a place that you could put the computer that meets two conditions? One, it is not in Steve's room so he's less tempted to use it past his bedtime. Two, it is some place in the house that is less noisy and distracting than the family room." They settled on putting the computer in the living room, which featured fewer distractions.

We also talked about frequency of computer usage. "This seems like a difficult situation. Steve says he needs to use the computer to do class assignments so it might be counterproductive to completely restrict his use of the computer. Should you establish some guidelines or rules for using the computer, though? For example, do you need to establish a firm bedtime? Do you limit amount of time spent in chat rooms? What would be helpful?" Steve and Ann established flexible guidelines that limited the amount of time on the computer, and they decided to implement them until Steve's next report card.

INFLUENCE OF INDIVIDUAL PSYCHOSOCIAL FACTORS

Self-Esteem and Locus of Control

Self-esteem and locus of control seem to be influenced by adolescent sexual behavior. Self-esteem seems to be influenced by congruity between values and behaviors: sexual behavior that contradicts personal values is associated with lower self-esteem and emotional distress (Miller, Christensen, and Olson, 1987). If an adolescent believes that sexual intercourse is acceptable and engages in intercourse, he or she is more likely to have high self-esteem. On the other hand, if an adolescent believes that sexual intercourse is unacceptable and engages in intercourse, he or she is more likely to have low self-esteem.

Stephanie Bowling discovered an interesting relationship between self-esteem and sexual behavior in focus groups she conducted to investigate influences of the father-daughter relationship on sexuality (Bowling and Werner-Wilson, 1998). Young women reported that self-esteem "definitely" influenced sexual behavior, but they were very clear that their relationship to their father significantly affected self-esteem. Locus of control also influences sexual attitudes of adolescent males (Werner-Wilson, 1998b).

This suggests that adolescents who engage in risky sexual behavior may be doing so because of low self-esteem or an external locus of control. They may seek affirmation or validation from others through sexual intimacy. If an adolescent client demonstrates low self-esteem or an external locus of control, one might want to inquire about sexual experimentation as well as quality of family support.

Religious Participation

Religious participation and locus of control were especially significant predictors of sexual attitudes for girls and boys (Werner-

Wilson, 1998b). "Religious *participation* was the most important predictor of sexual attitudes. Regular religious participation might provide the adolescent with a value system which, ostensibly, encouraged responsible sexual behavior—in the form of abstinence. Attendance at a house of worship might also provide the adolescent with regular social support and alternative activities to sexual experimentation" (Werner-Wilson, 1998b, p. 527). If these speculations are correct, there are clinical implications for family therapy: facilitate a discussion about values in therapy and encourage parents to provide social support. It might also be appropriate for adolescents to become involved in extracurricular school and/or community activities.

INFLUENCE OF DATING DYNAMICS

Adolescents who begin to date earlier have more dates, which is positively associated with (1) sexual experience; (2) number of sexual partners; and (3) level of sexual activity during later teen years (Miller, McCoy, and Olson, 1986; Thornton, 1990). Sexual experimentation at an early age is a positive predictor of sexual frequency. On the other hand, sexual experimentation at a later age is a positive predictor of safer sexual practices (Werner-Wilson and Vosburg, 1998).

Paradoxical Pregnancy

I consulted with the D family because the parents discovered that Lois, their fifteen-year-old daughter, was pregnant. Janet and Jerry, Lois' parents, identified themselves as "deeply religious." Jerry was a deacon at their church and Lois was also active in the congregation. All three identified as being "born-again Christian" and neither parents nor daughter considered abortion as an option because of these religious beliefs. In our initial session, Jerry was angry and accusatory. "How could you do this to yourself? How could you defile yourself and mock God and our beliefs?" Janet wept throughout the session and Lois seemed to have difficulty sustaining eye contact with anyone in the room. Lois expressed both shame and anger.

Donn Byrne (1977) published an article in *Psychology Today* titled "A Pregnant Pause in the Sexual Revolution" that seemed to address Lois' situation. Byrne's research suggested that both individual psychosocial factors and dating dynamics contribute to a phenomenon he identified as *paradoxical pregnancy.* Results from Bryne's study of young women at Indiana University suggested that participants who disapproved of premarital sex were less likely to use contraception. This belief paradoxically seemed to be associated with some of the women becoming pregnant: their disapproval reduced the likelihood that they would use contraception, so some who engaged in sexual intercourse became pregnant. Byrne referred to this as paradoxical pregnancy because the values of the young women were strong enough to inhibit using contraceptives but not strong enough to inhibit sexual experimentation. This phenomenon also places these young women at high risk for HIV/AIDS infection. Byrne suggested four possible explanations:

1. Avoidance of expectations that intercourse will occur reduces the likelihood that an adolescent will prepare for a sexual encounter.
2. Self-consciousness (adolescent egocentrism as discussed in Chapter 1) and a desire for privacy reduce the likelihood that an adolescent will take steps to obtain contraception.
3. Effective use of contraception requires regular attention and preparation, but adolescents who disapprove of sexual intercourse are less likely to consistently monitor contraceptive practices.
4. Adolescents who disapprove of sexual intercourse are less likely to talk to a partner about any aspect of sexuality, especially contraception.

The first three factors are primarily individual psychosocial factors, but the final one underscores the importance of communication in dating relationships. Communication about sexuality seems to be difficult for adolescents, particularly early in a dating relationship. This reluctance may be related to dating dynamics. Students report that being prepared for sexual intercourse early in a dating relationship is a social faux pas. Young men who prepare for sexual intercourse run the risk of offending their partner by "assuming" that their date is "easy," while women who prepare for intercourse run the risk of having their partner assume that they are sexually promiscuous. These tensions were exemplified during a recent class discussion between two students enrolled in a human sexuality class.

One young man commented, "If I take a condom out of my pocket, she'll be like, 'What kind of a girl do you think I am?'" to which a young woman replied, "And if I have a condom, he'll think that I'm a slut!"

Coercion

Coercion also influences dating dynamics. Social norms in the United States suggest that males should be sexually active, so they may pressure their partners to have sex. In some cases, this may lead to date rape. Some women, following an unwanted sexual encounter, may even blame themselves rather than their date. For example, I was consulting with Joan, a first-year university student, about her transition to living away from home for the first time. Not long after we began to work together, she made an appointment to see me earlier than our scheduled appointment. She sounded distraught.

Joan seemed composed when I met her in the waiting room but she began to cry as she sat down in her chair. "I've cheated on my fiancé and I *have* to tell him. I just know he'll break up with me."

"What happened?" I asked.

"I had sex with Bob last night. He's an old boyfriend. I wanted to have this extra session to help me figure out how to tell Steve."

"It might help if I knew a little bit more about what happened. Would you feel comfortable talking about it?"

Joan looked at the floor and answered in a hushed tone while tears streamed down her face. "Bob called last night and, like I told you, I've been feeling very alone on this campus. My roommate and I had gotten in another fight, so when Bob asked me to go for a pizza, I jumped at the chance. After we ate, we went back to his apartment and had sex."

I knew that Joan's fiancé, Steve, attended a university in another state. In an earlier session, Joan had told me that Bob had pushed to resume their relationship but that she wanted to remain friends with him, so I wondered about the possibility that Bob had coerced Joan into having sex. "What happened at the restaurant?" I asked.

"Our waiter was really slow so it took us forever to get our order. Bob was telling jokes and being silly while we were waiting. We were having fun." Joan stopped crying as she related details of the evening.

"Did you have anything to drink?" I asked.

"Yeah. We had a couple of pitchers. Like I said, the waiter was slow so we had plenty of time to kill."

"How much beer did you have? A glass, a couple of glasses, a pitcher?"

"Well, we had two pitchers and I drank at least as much as Bob so I guess I had a pitcher or so."

"Did you drive or did Bob?"

"Bob did. Now that I think about it, he didn't drink as much as me because he said he was driving. He told me to relax, that he'd take care of me."

"What happened when you went to Bob's apartment?" I asked.

"That part's kind of fuzzy. I think I told him to take me home but he said that I shouldn't be alone. He told me that we'd have more fun at his place." She resumed crying. "Then we had sex and now I've wrecked my engagement."

"If this is too embarrassing or painful to talk about right now, we can talk about something else." I paused. "But I would like to know what happened after you went back to Bob's apartment."

"Well, I was feeling kind of sick so we sat down. He turned on some music, I think. Then he started to kiss me and the next thing I know he's on top of me."

"Did you pass out, Joan? You said that he started to kiss you and the next thing you knew he was on top of you. Did you pass out between the kiss and him getting on top of you?"

"Yeah, I guess I did."

"Did you ask Bob to stop?"

"Yeah, I think I did. Yes, I did. When I woke up I told him to stop. He told me to shut up and then he put it in and, and. . . ." Joan began to sob. She had interpreted this event as an act of unfaithfulness and blamed herself for having sex with Bob when he had encouraged her to drink more beer, persuaded her to go to his apartment, and ignored her plea to stop. Joan seemed to blame herself for being victimized by someone who engaged in sexual coercion.

In cases where young women disapprove of premarital sexual intercourse, they may violate their own standards because of a partner's insistence. In these cases, sexual coercion is more subtle but still devastating. I supervised a case at a campus clinic in which a young woman initiated therapy because of academic difficulties. She told her therapist that she lacked motivation to attend her classes and, when she did attend, had difficulty paying attention to class lectures. She also reported that she had fallen behind on class assignments. The student had earned a 3.5 grade point average in her first year at the university, so the therapist inquired about relationships.

The student confided in her therapist that she had been feeling "miserable" since she broke up with her boyfriend. "We were supposed to get married after we graduated but he decided that he didn't love me anymore." The couple had dated for three years and, at some point during the second year of the relationship, they began to have intercourse.

"I figured that after two years we might as well have sex. After all, we had done pretty much everything else so why not intercourse? I thought it would be okay since he said he loved me and we were engaged to be married. He told me that he already considered us married since we were 'soul mates' so it didn't make sense to wait. I had wanted to wait until after I was married to do it, but I got tired of him always bringing it up." This young woman told her therapist that she felt "dirty, used, and ashamed."

INFLUENCE OF FAMILY RELATIONSHIPS

Parents often fear that their influence is less important than peer influence. Research suggests, though, that the strength of peer influence on sexuality is mediated by parent-adolescent communication (Wright, Peterson, and Barnes, 1990). Although young college women rate friends, schools, and books as more important than parents as *sources* of information about sex, parents are rated as having more influence on sexual attitudes (Sanders and Mullis, 1988). Similarly, in a study of 1,551 high school students, there was a correlation between virginity and parental encouragement for abstinence: virgins and girls reported that they cared more about their parents' feelings than what a boyfriend or girlfriend thought (Jenson, DeGaston, and Weed, 1994).

Sexual permissiveness about intercourse is related to parental discipline and control: democratic parenting has the strongest influence (Miller et al., 1986). In a recent study by Werner-Wilson (1998b) the second best predictor of adolescent boys' sexual attitudes was fathers' attitudes about adolescent intercourse (as previously mentioned, religious participation was the most significant predictor). In the same study, adolescent girls were influenced by mothers' attitudes about adolescent sexual intercourse, parental discussion of sexual values, and general communication with fathers.

Parent support of sex education is negatively associated with adolescent pregnancy: adolescent females who discussed sexuality with their parents were less likely to become pregnant (Murry, 1992), and sex education workshops that featured parent and adolescent participation reduced the likelihood of pregnancy (Postrado and Nicholson, 1992). Despite the ability to influence adolescent contraception use, parents seemed unlikely to be supportive of sex education because they lacked knowledge and understanding about human sexuality (Jorgensen, 1981). Parent participation in sexuality education is discussed in the following section.

Parents also indirectly influence adolescent sexuality. For example, a longitudinal study of seventy-six seventh-grade girls and their parents revealed that parent distance is positively associated with symptoms of depression in females; these symptoms are positively associated with sexually permissive attitudes and friends who are sexually active (Whitbeck, Conger, and Kao, 1993). Sibling relationships are also associated with adolescent sexual activity. Earlier sexual experience is positively correlated with older siblings who are sexually active (Hogan and Kitagawa, 1985); this may occur due to role modeling (East, Felice, and Morgan, 1993), or it may result from greater parental permissiveness (Rodgers, Rowe, and Harris, 1992).

PARENTAL INVOLVEMENT
IN SEXUALITY EDUCATION

Given the research evidence that, despite the fact that parents fundamentally influence the sexuality of adolescents, parents are reluctant to become involved in the sexuality education process, our research team conducted focus group interviews with adolescents and their parents. The material in this section is based on a presentation titled "How Can Mothers and Fathers Become Involved in the Sexuality Education of Adolescents?" (Werner-Wilson and Coughlin-Smith, 1997) given at the National Council on Family Relations. This research has an important bearing on family therapy that seeks to enhance communication between parents and teens about sexuality, so this particular project is discussed in depth.

Sample and Research Procedure

We conducted focus group interviews with participants from two communities in southwest Michigan. We focused, for the present study, on data from two questions: "What should be done to help teenagers reduce risky sexual practices?" and "What needs to be done to increase condom use among teenagers who are sexually active?"

We employed a snowball sample to recruit participants: we asked each person who agreed to participate to provide us with the names of other families who might be willing to participate in our study. We interviewed adolescent girls and their families as well as adolescent boys and their families at each site. Separate interviews were conducted with each member of the family, so we have data from interviews with two groups of girls ($n = 8$), boys ($n = 6$), mothers of girls ($n = 7$), mothers of boys ($n = 5$), fathers of girls ($n = 6$), and fathers of boys ($n = 5$).

The average age for girls was fifteen and the average age for boys was sixteen. Although all of the adolescent participants indicated on the anonymous questionnaire that they were virgins, most of them ($n = 13$) had friends who had experienced sexual intercourse. Additionally, all of the adolescents indicated that they were "exclusively heterosexual." The majority (71 percent) of the adolescents lived with both biological parents and annual family income ranged from $30,000 to $70,000. The average family income for participants was $60,000.

What Should Be Done to Help Teenagers Reduce Risky Sexual Practices?

Adolescent Males

Adolescent males suggested that education—including consequences of sexual behavior (e.g., unintended pregnancy and STDs) and technical aspects of different contraceptive methods—was the primary method to reduce risky sexual behaviors. One adolescent, for example, suggested that "[health educators] should show you different contraceptives and how you could use them." They provided three topics for consideration: (1) sexual restraint; (2) specific information about STDs; and (3) response to sexual coercion.

Adolescent Females

Adolescent females, rather than focusing on topics of conversation, focused on aspects of relationships that facilitate communication about sexuality. They reported that they wanted to discuss sexuality with someone they trusted, but suggested that they were reluctant to talk to their parents because they perceived that their parents would be judgmental: "I wouldn't go to my parents or an adult because I know they're strongly against having sex"; ". . . if you have a problem you usually don't go to your parents"; "We need someone who can be honest with us without stating a direct opinion." Friends and siblings were common sources of information. One participant, for example, described discussing sexuality with her brother: "Actually, it's easier talking to him than some of my friends." She suggested that he was more likely to be honest with her.

Mothers

Mothers also recognized the need to have an open dialogue with their children: "I think the biggest part is you have to be honest with them so that they feel they can come and talk to you." Despite this recommendation, adolescent females' perception that their parents were judgmental may be linked to mothers' suggestion that risky sexual practices would be reduced by focusing on values: ". . . I think we have to build responsibility and look at our values." Mothers also suggested the following: (1) monitor adolescents' behavior; (2) attend to their own behaviors as role models; (3) become involved in sexuality education; and (4) support sexuality education at schools. The following examples reflect monitoring suggestions: "Don't let them [participate] in situations that are . . . uncontrolled" and "And curfew. You don't stay out all night. That's when you get into trouble." One mother suggested her influence as a role model was lifelong: ". . . and just being good role models from the very beginning as they're toddlers and just growing up with you." Mothers seemed to have some ambivalence about sexuality education. On one hand, they suggested that it should occur at home but they also recognized the importance of having it presented at school. As one mother noted, ". . . a lot of the parents don't want to do it. I'd rather have it done at home, but there are a lot of kids out there just experimenting."

Fathers

Fathers recommended three strategies to reduce risky behavior: (1) monitor external influences such as peers and the media; (2) encourage abstinence; and (3) promote education in the home and in the classroom. Fathers, concerned about peer influence, suggested that parents should regulate "who they're running around with or who they're with. If they're constantly with kids that are sexually active, then I assume they're gonna be sexually active." Fathers' perceptions about sexuality education in schools seemed to be compatible with those of adolescent males: "The kids need information . . . presented in a factual way, not necessarily in an emotional way. They need to know the pros and cons and it needs to be presented in a manner that they will accept." One father saw it as an important paternal responsibility: "It's my obligation as a parent; comfortable or not, I need to talk about it at least some. And if I can't do it, then I need to find someone else as a parent that could."

What Needs to Be Done to Increase Condom Use Among Teenagers Who Are Sexually Active?

Adolescent Males

Adolescent males focused primarily on availability of condoms. Increased access, it was suggested, would result in more frequent condom use. Adolescent males provided several recommendations to increase access, but they also noted that if condoms were more readily available "parents would get angry because they don't want schools to do that." They suggested two strategies: (1) help adolescents become more comfortable purchasing condoms at retail stores; and (2) make condoms more available at school.

Adolescent Females

Adolescent females also addressed availability of condoms but there was disagreement about condom dispensers in schools. One exchange between participants reflects support for distribution in schools: "I think schools should hand them out. . . ." "There are so many kids having sex," and "They're, like, embarrassed to go to the store and buy them. . . ." One adolescent female summarized this position: "It's [condom dispensers in schools] saying, if you're gonna do it, at least do it safely. It's *not* saying, 'OK, I want all of you to go out and have sex now because there's a condom machine in the bathroom.'" This point of view was not, however, unanimous: "If you have one [a condom] just to be like the rest of your friends, then maybe you bring it into your home and your younger siblings find it." Adolescent girls, in addition to discussing availability of condoms, also suggested that television could help promote condom use. One participant, for example, suggested "going with it [an advertisement] as a kid's point of view."

Mothers

Mothers seemed divided in their perceptions about condom use. Some indicated that the topic should be discussed while others feared that availability of condoms promoted premarital sexual experimentation. One mother suggested, "If the parents don't promote the use of contraceptives, if the kids are afraid of getting caught using contraceptives, then they won't use them. Then you're gonna have, you know, worse consequences." In support, a second mother noted, "I used to think that having condoms available for young children and students was wrong, but that's when I thought the world was black and white." One mother feared that an abstinence-only approach was dangerous: "The reality of it is that in the heat of the moment, [the idea] that abstinence is the best thing doesn't enter into the situation at all. So we really haven't given them any tools to use in reality." There was disagreement: "I have a real problem with that . . . abstinence until marriage is the way we're raising our children and to promote condom use goes against that." Another noted, "I'm not encouraging my kid to use condoms; I'm encouraging him not to use them." Mothers who discussed condom use with their children recommended direct communication: "And I said, 'I don't expect you to carry them, please, but if that ever comes up I would expect you to do that.' "

Fathers

Fathers also disagreed about promoting condom use. Like mothers, some feared that encouraging condom use would be interpreted as tacit encouragement for sexual experimentation: "I don't know if I want to increase their use because then . . . you're gonna have to increase their sexual activity" and "My opinion is that they need to know that there are contraceptives. I believe that students, if they choose to and the situation is correct, correct for them in their minds, are going to have sex. . . . If they are going to have sex, I surely want them to know about contraception." Fathers struggled to provide specific suggestions, but they did suggest that appeals based on fear were unlikely to have an impact on teenagers: "I think the more intelligent that a kid is, the more scare tactics really just kinda turn them off."

Recommendations

How can mothers and fathers become involved in the sexuality education of adolescents? Parental involvement is likely to be difficult because parents and adolescents disagree about fundamental issues. More often than not, adolescents provide specific strategies for reducing risky sexual practices and encouraging condom use. Parents, however, seem to have difficulty embracing the sexuality of adolescents, so they seem to have difficulty developing specific recommendations. Data from adolescents provide us with some clues for parent involvement:

- Parents could cultivate an atmosphere of respect for adolescent behavior.
- Parents could listen, rather than lecture, to concerns about sexuality raised by adolescent children.

- Parents could provide support and factual information.
- Parents could help their adolescent children respond to sexual coercion by talking to children about dating and expectations.

Many parents who participated in our focus groups told us that talking about the topic in a group with other parents helped relieve anxiety and provided them with the incentive to take a more active role in discussing sex with their children. Family therapy with adolescents and their parents can provide a forum for similar discussions. If families accept this invitation, these discusions should be structured to promote open dialogue about influences such as media, self-esteem, technical material, and values. It may be particularly important to address sexual coercion, social double standards, and family support. I use variations of the following "starter" questions to help families have these discussions:

- How is intimacy and affection expressed in your family? What are your specific needs and how can other family members help meet these needs?
- What could your parents do to help you feel safe talking about sex?
- How could you become more comfortable initiating a conversation about sex with your children?
- How could _____ (adolescent child) talk to you about sexual coercion in a relationship without you forbidding him or her to date an individual?
- How can you have a conversation about sex that addresses values without it turning into a lecture?
- How can you become comfortable talking to _____ (adolescent child) about your own sexual experiences?

Accepting responsibility for initiating these discussions may be difficult. Talking about sex is not easy for families or for therapists so comfort zones may need to be expanded when talking about sex. Before initiating discussions with families, it may be helpful for therapists to assess their own values and prejudices about adolescent sexuality in order to make them transparent to their clients.

Making this effort on behalf of one's clients may help them openly discuss an important but avoided aspect of our humanity.

SUMMARY

Adolescents are naturally curious about sexuality and this review of research suggests that parents are a primary source of influence on adolescent sexual attitudes and behavior, but parents seem uncomfortable openly discussing these topics. Given parent reluctance, one might want to invite families to discuss sexuality.

Chapter 9

Alcohol and Substance Abuse

Adolescents may experience problems related to alcohol and substance abuse in two ways: *personal misuse* and *parental misuse.* Increasingly, treatment of alcohol and substance abuse includes treatment of family members. In this chapter I review trends associated with adolescent alcohol and substance abuse and discuss conceptual issues associated with treatment. I detail a treatment approach that relies on a structural approach to family therapy.

TRENDS

Joseph A. Califano Jr. and Alyse Booth (1998) of the National Center on Addiction and Substance Abuse (CASA) at Columbia University reported the following key findings related to the "drug-plagued world of our teens" (p. 8):

- Teens rate drugs as the single most important problem.
- Teens report easy access to illegal substances: 45 percent of high school students say they could purchase marijuana in an hour or less and only 14 percent report that they would not know how to obtain it.

Developmental Components

Findings from Califano and Booth (1998) suggest that there are developmental influences on use of illegal substances. For example, 16 percent of twelve- to fourteen-year-olds have personally seen drugs sold on school grounds, but 37 percent of older teens have witnessed a drug transaction on school property. Califano and Booth identify the transition from age twelve to age thirteen as a "turning point" associated with exposure to illegal substances:

- The proportion of teens who say they could purchase marijuana if they wanted to triples from 14 percent to 50 percent.
- The percentage of teens who report that they know someone who sells illegal substances increases from 8 percent to 22 percent.
- Fewer older teens (85 percent) than younger teens (52 percent) are willing to report a fellow student whom they personally saw using illegal substances.

Family Influence on Adolescent Use of Alcohol and Illegal Substances

Two recent national studies report that family relationships have a significant influence on adolescents' use of alcohol and illegal substances. Michael Resnick and his colleagues from the Adolescent Health Program at the University of Minnesota surveyed more than 12,000 adolescents in grades seven through twelve. Resnick and his colleagues (1997) report that adolescents are less likely to use alcohol or marijuana if (1) there is frequent interaction with their parents, and (2) they experience a high degree of connectedness with their parents.

The Califano and Booth (1998) report and another report from CASA highlight the importance of parental involvement. According to their 1998 study, adolescents who regularly eat dinner with their parents are less likely to abuse illegal substances. A second study (National Center on Addiction and Substance Abuse at Columbia University, 1999a) reports that father involvement seems to be particularly important. Adolescents who report that they have only a fair or poor relationship with their father are at much greater risk (68 percent) for smoking, drinking, or using illegal substances. Califano, who is a former U.S. Secretary of Health, Education, and Welfare, concluded, "This is a wake-up call for every dad in America. . . . It's time for every father in America to look in the mirror and ask: How often do I eat meals with my children? Take them to religious services? Help with their homework? Attend their games and extracurricular activities? Join mom in monitoring my teen's conduct, praising and disciplining them?" (National Center on Addiction and Substance Abuse at Columbia University, 1999b).

Effect of Parent Misuse of Alcohol or Illegal Substances

Alcohol and substance abuse is not only a problem for adolescents, it is also a problem when parents of adolescents misuse substances. Jeanne Reid, Peggy Macchetto, and Susan Foster (1999) of CASA surveyed more than 900 social service professionals to measure their perception of problems associated with substance abuse. They report the following key findings:

- Substance abuse causes or exacerbates 70 percent of cases of child abuse or neglect.
- Children whose parents abuse alcohol or illegal substances are three times more likely to abuse and four times more likely to be neglected than children whose parents do not abuse alcohol or illegal substances.
- Most (71.6 percent) of the social service providers conclude that abuse of alcohol and illegal substances is one of the main reasons that there has been an increase in the mistreatment of children.

Reid and colleagues also conducted case studies on the effect of alcohol and substance abuse on children and adolescents. One sixteen-year-old describes living with a parent who is a substance abuser: "It's awful in the long run . . . when you grow up to have to deal with a lot more problems, 'cause when you're little you don't realize everything that's happening, and you try to understand and you don't. And then you get older, it's so hard to think that your mom would do that to you. I mean she'll tell you that she loves you and that she'll help you in any way she can—but she doesn't. She tries but she can't; the drugs take over. And I don't know, it's just hard. It's really hard" (Reid, Machetto, and Foster, 1999, p. 3).

TREATMENT OF ALCOHOL AND SUBSTANCE ABUSE: CONCEPTUAL ISSUES

Donald Davis (1987) developed an integrative approach to alcohol and substance abuse that is based on the premise that family interactional processes maintain alcohol or substance abuse. He contends that all aspects of family life are influenced by problem drinking:

- Marital satisfaction is negatively influenced.
- Communication is impaired.
- Alcoholism or substance abuse is associated with partner abuse, and physical and sexual abuse of children.
- Children of parents who abuse alcohol or other substances suffer emotionally (e.g., they may accept responsibility for parenting their parents).
- Children of parents who abuse alcohol or other substances often experience difficulty establishing and maintaining intimate relationships.
- Children of parents who abuse alcohol or other substances may be predisposed to experience a substance abuse problem.

M. Duncan Stanton and colleagues (1982) developed one of the first approaches to treatment that incorporated family therapy. In their conceptual model, they suggested that alcohol and substance abuse problems originate during adolescence. They contend that experimentation with alcohol is a normal part of adolescence and that early use is primarily social in nature. Adolescents are at highest risk for abusing alcohol or drugs if they have problematic relationships with their family.

This conceptualization features a developmental component that has significant implications for treatment. First, if the adolescent is the family member who is abusing alcohol or substances, this model suggests assessing quality of family relationships and addressing these aspects in treatment. If the parent is the family member who is abusing alcohol or other substances, recognize that the problem may be a long-standing one. If, as Stanton suggests, misuse develops because of problems in adolescence, then recognize that it may be firmly entrenched as a coping mechanism for the particular individual.

Both of these clinical conceptualizations are consistent with results from the surveys discussed earlier. The research, then, provides empirical support for these conceptual approaches.

Functions of Alcohol and Substance Abuse

Most approaches to treatment have recognized that alcohol and substance abuse serve a function for families. Donald Davis (1987) suggested the following propositions:

1. Abuse of alcohol or other substances has adaptive consequences.
2. The adaptive consequences reinforce abuse.
3. Primary factors for each individual are different. Intrapsychic phenomena, couple dynamics, family relationships, or larger systems may influence alcohol or substance abuse.

Stanton and his colleagues described the functions of alcohol and substance abuse in terms of family cycles. They suggest that addiction is influenced by "a complex set of feedback mechanisms within a repetitive cycle" (Stanton et al., 1982, p. 22). In the case of adolescent alcohol or substance abuse, problem behaviors distract parents from other family problems (e.g., marital conflict):

1. When family equilibrium is threatened, the addict creates a situation that focuses on her or him.
2. After the family crisis subsides, the addict begins to behave more competently.
3. As the addict begins to act more competently, conflict increases in other parts of the family. This perpetuates the cycle.

Assessment

Stanton and his colleagues identified several features of families that include a member who is abusing alcohol or other substances. These features could be part of a clinical assessment:

- There is a higher frequency of multigenerational chemical dependency.
- Families of addicts seem to be more primitive and direct in their expression of conflict.

- Alliances are more explicit.
- Addicts' families feature a "preponderance" of death themes and premature or untimely deaths.
- Addiction serves the purpose of false differentiation.

David W. Brook and Judith S. Brook (1992) have investigated family processes associated with alcohol and drug abuse. These factors could also be used for clinical assessment. They identified the following family characteristics that correlate with adolescent drug use:

1. Relative lack of parental supervision
2. Weak parent-child mutual attachment
3. Conflictual relationship between parent and adolescent
4. Family tolerance for deviant, illegal, or unconventional behavior
5. Family members who abuse alcohol or other substances
6. Family members who are unconventional, aggressive, or socially isolated
7. Parental psychopathology or poverty
8. Parental divorce, death, or abandonment

The Family Assessment Device (discussed in Chapter 6) could be used to screen for possible alcohol or substance abuse. For example, problems associated with communication or affective involvement could lead the therapist to inquire about alcohol or substance abuse.

In cases where one might want to supplement clinical evaluation, an instrument has been developed that seems to be a useful screening tool. Melvin L. Selzer developed the Michigan Alcoholism Screening Test (MAST), which has been widely used in research and clinical practice to measure alcoholism. Measuring alcohol and substance abuse is often difficult because respondents may not be truthful, but the MAST was designed to address this problem. It has proven to be both reliable and clinically useful. There are two versions of the test. The long version (Selzer, 1971) includes twenty-four items, and the short version (Selzer, Vinokur, and van Rooijen, 1975) includes thirteen questions.

Treatment Models

Most contemporary treatment models of alcohol and substance abuse are based on a multidimensional approach. Each of the following texts on treatment incorporates multiple models of therapy for treatment:

> Davis, D. I. (1987). *Alcoholism treatment: An integrative family and individual approach.* New York: Gardner Press.[1]

> Kaufman, E. and Kaufmann, P. (Eds.). (1992). *Family therapy of drug and alcohol abuse* (Second edition). New York: Allyn and Bacon.[2]

> Lawson, A. and Lawson, G. (1998). *Alcoholism and the family: A guide to treatment and prevention* (Second edition). Gaithersburg, Maryland: Aspen Publishers.[3]

> Stanton, M. D. and Todd, T. C. (Eds.). (1982). *The family therapy of drug abuse and addiction.* New York: Guilford Press.[4]

The discussion of emotional development (Chapter 2) covered the major principles associated with Bowenian family systems therapy and symbolic experiential therapy, so those models will not be elaborated on in this chapter. There is a significant amount of redundancy among behavioral, strategic, and structural models of family therapy, so only one of these approaches to alcohol and substance abuse will be reviewed. Structural family therapy will be discussed because it seems to be incorporated in more treatment models and includes aspects of the other two models. It also includes features of treatment that are consistent with experiential and Bowenian models.

TREATMENT OF ALCOHOL AND SUBSTANCE ABUSE: STRUCTURAL FAMILY THERAPY

Structural family therapy incorporates ideas that are consistent with developmental psychology, symbolic experiential therapy, social constructionism, family development theory, and solution-focused therapy. Family therapists Salvador Minuchin and Howard Fishman in their book *Family Therapy Techniques* (1981) note that therapists become a part of the family system during therapy and suggest that use of self facilitates this process. Both of these ideas are consistent with symbolic experiential family therapy (see Chapter 11 by Robert Marrs on use of self in therapy) and social constructionist approaches to family therapy (see Chapter 12 by Darren Wozny).

Minuchin and Fishman also incorporate ideas from a family development perspective and suggest that aspects of adolescent development fundamentally affect family dynamics. As a child becomes an adolescent, Minuchin and Fishman suggest that issues of autonomy and control must be renegotiated on *all levels* (adolescents' need for both connection and independence is discussed further in Chapters 5 and 6).

In cases of alcohol or substance abuse, the family often organizes around the drinking or use of illegal drugs. During the initial stage of therapy, the family and therapist form a partnership that features three therapeutic goals:

1. Free the family symptom bearer of a symptom
   (in this case, alcohol or substance abuse).
2. Reduce conflict and stress for the whole family.
3. Help the family learn new ways of coping.

Minuchin and Fishman suggest that treatment planning is a crucial part of therapy process and describe several types of families and typical problems associated with each type. Their description of *out-of-control* families is relevant to this discussion of alcohol and substance abuse. These families often have multiple members who have symptoms (e.g., both parent and adolescent are problem drinkers or are substance abusers). In addition to the three general goals associated with therapy, Minuchin and Fishman identify two other family structure goals for these families:

1. Promote structure in which parents accept responsibility
   for executive functions.
2. Promote cohesive communication.

Minuchin and Fishman suggest three approaches to facilitate change: (1) *challenge the symptom*, (2) *challenge the family structure*, or (3) *challenge the family reality*. *Challenge* is used to refer to the search for new interactional patterns and "does not imply harsh maneuvers, or confrontation, though at times both may be indicated" (Minuchin and Fishman, 1981, p. 67).

Challenge the Symptom

Rather than focus exclusively on "curing" a symptom, we want to challenge the family's perception that the symptom is the problem. When looking for an opportunity to challenge symptoms of alcohol or substance abuse, observe family interactional patterns to identify ineffective but repetitive patterns. To borrow an idea from strategic family therapy, attempted solutions (the interaction pattern) contribute to the maintenance of the problem (alcohol or substance abuse behaviors). The goal is to change or reframe the family's view of the problem by directly or indirectly challenging the nature of the familial response to the problem. Three specific techniques are recommended: *enactment, focusing,* and *increasing intensity.*

Enactment

An enactment is an intervention that provides important information about interactional patterns. One way to do this is to take advantage of opportunities as they are presented in therapy. For example, if a family begins to argue about something, encourage them to continue arguing rather than attempt to mediate the dispute. Clients may expect therapists to stop a conflict or to facilitate a shared understanding, but when using enactment to challenge the system, the therapist wants to observe the patterns rather than intervene. Instead of mediating, the therapist shares observations about the influence of particular interaction patterns (e.g., rescuing, forming coalitions, changing the subject) in order to challenge the symptom.

Focusing

The technique of focusing helps to challenge the symptom by attending to particular themes or interactional patterns in a systematic manner that permits examination of one small theme in depth. Use focusing to develop a structural goal and a strategy to achieve it. For example, challenge enmeshed patterns that help facilitate alcohol or substance abuse in a family by focusing on ways to encourage more independence in relationships.

Increasing Intensity

Raising intensity is another method therapists use to challenge the symptom. One way to raise intensity is to use repetition. Therapists can increase intensity dramatically by using repetition to facilitate focus. This is particularly effective for families that engage in "hit-and-run" attacks on one another. During an enactment, simply observe these attacks, but when seeking to raise intensity, focus on the pattern. Point it out to the family and ask them to respond to it. This would help demonstrate ways in which the symptom is maintained by interaction patterns.

Challenge Family Structure

In addition to challenging the symptom, change can be facilitated by challenging family coalitions (structures) that help maintain alcohol or substance abuse. Flexibility is an asset to families. The goal is to change relationship coalitions that exist between family members in order to permit alternative ways of thinking and feeling. Minuchin and Fishman suggest two problems associated with level of closeness in relationships: *enmeshment* (overaffiliation) and *disengagement* (underaffiliation).

Family structure can be assessed by paying attention to seating arrangements and interactional patterns. If two parents attend therapy, where do they sit in proximity to each other? For example, if a child consistently sits between her or his parents, we may wonder if the child is used as a buffer between the adults. Alternatively, parents might systematically sit away from each other and next to a particular child. This might suggest a coalition.

Interactional patterns provide additional information to us about family structure. Examples of enmeshed communication include:

- Interruptions that disrupt an individual's personal experience
- Finishing sentences for other family members
- Interpreting other's feelings or intentions (e.g., "What he really means is . . .")

Examples of disengaged communication include:

- Ignoring what a family member is saying. Rather than making eye contact and encouraging someone else to talk, in a disengaged relationship the nonspeaking person may pay attention to objects in the office or simply stare blankly into space.
- Introducing an unrelated topic. Rather than addressing a topic previously discussed, there is a pattern in which different family members drift off into different topics of personal relevance.

Minuchin and Fishman recommend three tactics to facilitate challenges to the family structure: *boundary making, unbalancing,* and *teaching complementarity.*

Boundary Making

Techniques of boundary making are designed to provide more flexibility in relationships. It is desirable to support both connectedness and separation. To this end, try to facilitate different closeness levels by rearranging physical space (e.g., asking family members to move to other seats). Support boundary making by assigning tasks that facilitate different forms of interaction (e.g., asking a parent who is disengaged from a particular child to perform some mutual activity with that child). Finally, cultivate clear boundaries between the therapist and the family.

Unbalancing

Boundary making techniques can change levels of closeness between family members. Unbalancing techniques are used to address family organization (e.g., hierarchical structure). We can unbalance relationships by alternating our affiliation with family members, ignoring a particular family member or coalition for a particular period of time, or forming a coalition against a family member or coalition. Use of self is an important part of this process because

> the therapist will have to use herself, as a member of the therapeutic system, to challenge and change the family power allocation. Family members expect the therapist to be "firm but fair." . . . Instead, the therapist joins and supports one individual or one subsystem at the expense of the others. She affiliates with a family member low in a hierarchy, empowering him instead of undercutting him. (Minuchin and Fishman, 1981, p. 161)

Teaching Complementarity

Family structure can also be changed by encouraging family members to become more complementary in their relationships. Therapists want to help family members be competent in participating in a full range of human experiences. This helps to reduce restricted, rigid roles. One way to accomplish this is to expand the family's view of the problem. By examining the function of alcohol or substance abuse in the family and the ways in which family relationships actually reinforce abuse, properties of family structure are addressed. This also supports the process of challenging the symptom in the family.

Challenge Family Reality

In Chapter 12, Darren Wozny describes the benefits of adopting a postmodern, social constructionist approach to therapy with adolescents and their families. Harvey Joanning (1992), who completed federally funded research on adolescent substance abuse, has suggested that this approach is helpful in treating alcohol and substance abuse. Structural family therapy refers to this as *challenging the family reality.* Reality is based on "the meaning we give to the aggregate of facts that we recognize as facts. And there is one more step. Reality has to be shared with others—others who validate it" (Minuchin and Fishman, 1981, p. 209). There are three main categories that relate to family reality: *universal symbols, family truths,* and *expert advice.*

Rigid perceptions of reality can be challenged by incorporating universal symbols in therapy. This includes using ideas based on "common sense" understandings of behavior or relationships or ideas based on larger forces such as cultural norms. These universal symbols influence family truths: "The therapist pays attention to the family's justifications of their transactions and uses their same worldview to expand their functioning" (Minuchin and Fishman, 1981, p. 227). Although reality is a social construction, therapists can relate their clinical experience or expertise in a particular area to help expand family reality by providing expert advice.

SUMMARY

Alcohol and substance abuse create problems for adolescents and their families when parents abuse these substances and/or when adolescents abuse them. Family dynamics seem to influence adolescent abuse and many family therapy approaches rely on principles of structural family therapy.

Chapter 10

Suicide

Darren A. Wozny

One of parents' worst fears is learning that their adolescent is considering suicide or has already attempted it. Even if conflict in the family is not overt, feelings of betrayal may exist. For the adolescent struggling with suicidal thoughts, there are overtones of a disconnection from the very people that could help most: parents, siblings, peers, teachers, and others. This particular "family in crisis" presents a daunting challenge to family therapists who must deal not only with emotionally charged family members and often distraught adolescents, but also their own reactions.

The primary premise of this chapter is that the issue of suicide among adolescents and their families creates a "pressure cooker" context that often prevents the kinds of relational support that protect the family from the premature exit of its young members. It is through the therapist's ongoing caring relationship with the adolescent and the family that a context of hopefulness and support becomes the prime growing condition for more preferred and protective family relationships.

RESEARCH ON SUICIDE AND ADOLESCENCE

Before introducing the individual risk factors, I would like to discuss suicide from a macro perspective. This is pertinent to therapists because in planning clinical services it gives a rough estimate of the kinds of issues a clinician is likely to encounter. In the United States, there are approximately 30,000 suicide deaths per year, almost eighty-three per day. There are three million nonfatal suicide attempt injuries per year. Combined, these figures amount to more than 8,300 suicide behaviors a day, or approximately 346 per hour (Ramsey et al., 1993).

Any family therapist who works regularly with adolescents and their families will frequently encounter the issue of suicide. Suicide is the third leading cause of death in the adolescent age range of fifteen to twenty-four years. Currently, 20 percent of all male suicides and 14 percent of all female suicides come from this age group (Stevenson, 1988).

RISK FACTORS

It is important for the clinician to be aware of high-risk groups for suicide so that in initial assessments therapists can invite some conversation to ensure that suicide is not involved.

Completed suicides are three-and-a-half times more common among males than females (Ramsey et al., 1993; Stevenson, 1988). One plausible explanation is that half of the completed suicides by males occur using firearms, which have a low chance of rescue and recovery. Young women, however, are four to five times more likely to engage in suicide attempts than young men. The most common suicide method employed by females is overdosing, which allows a window of time for a change of intent, as well as the chance of rescue and recovery (Ramsey et al., 1993).

Several studies have shown that gay and lesbian adolescents are up to six times more likely to attempt suicide than a comparable control group of unmarried heterosexual adolescents (Bell and Weinberg, 1978; Saghir and Robins, 1973; Jay and Young, 1979; Marten et al., 1985). Ramsey and colleagues (1993) pointed out that records of completed suicide often do not contain information on sexual orientation; therefore, the risk of completed suicide for this population ranges from three to seventeen times more than the heterosexual controls.

Gay men are more likely to attempt suicide in their adolescent years when they are trying to "come out." Lesbian women's attempts occur at a later age and are more commonly related to break up of relationships (Ramsey et al., 1993). Gay and lesbian adolescents considering suicide may experience particular difficulty finding social support due to the prevalence of homophobic attitudes.

Though the rates of suicide among young African-American men are lower than those of their Caucasian counterparts, the rate has risen threefold over the last twenty-five years, tripling for African-American males and doubling for African-American females (Ramsey et al., 1993; Centers for Disease Control, 1985). Suicide rates for Hispanic populations are lower than both Caucasians or African-Americans, and most often occur in the age group of twenty to twenty-four with Hispanic men (Ramsey et al., 1993; Centers for Disease Control, 1985).

Careful consideration is required prior to using antidepressant medication to treat a patient who has a history of suicide attempt by overdose. Several studies have suggested that the use of tricyclic antidepressants are associated with a higher suicide rate, possibly because of the lethality of these agents in overdose, their relative ineffectiveness in treating youthful mood disorders, or their tendency to be prescribed for youth at high risk for suicide (Brent et al., 1993; Kapur, Mieczkowski, and Mann, 1992; Pfeffer et al., 1994). In cases of suicide risk, selective serotonergic reuptake inhibitors are preferable to tricyclic antidepressants. Selective serotonergic reuptake inhibitors apparently carry a lower risk of suicide and suicide attempts (Kapur, Mieczkowski, and Mann, 1992; Brent, 1997).

One study found that suicidal clients who had twenty-four-hour backup from a physician had lower rates of suicidal behavior (Morgan, Jones, and Owen, 1993). I would recommend physician involvement, especially if the adolescent is on medication; and in cases where medications are not involved, a primary physician may be instrumental should hospitalization become warranted.

Individual Risk Factors

Membership of adolescents in one of the previously identified high risk-groups is not sufficient in estimating the immediate risk for self-harm. Discussion must address the suicide intent inherent in the current suicide plan, exploration of previous history of suicide attempts, and protective resources.

Suicide intent refers to the extent that the adolescent wishes to die. Suicide intent is quite slippery because the intuitive relationship between level of self-harm and suicide intent is not what one would expect. This seems related to Brent's (1997) finding that the lethality of the intent, or medical damage, is only modestly associated with suicidal intent. It is problematic to rely primarily on the adolescent's self-report of suicidal intent, therefore it is necessary to look for outward indicators of dangerous intent.

Items that discriminate between completers and attempters and are presumably related to high suicide intent include the following: evidence of planning, timing the attempt to avoid detection, confiding suicide plans ahead of time, and expressing a wish to die (Brent, 1997).

Contrary to common belief, suicide rarely occurs without warning. Beskow (1979) indicated that upwards of 80 percent of those who have completed suicide have communicated to others their intent to commit the act. Adam (1985) reports that a primary characteristic of nearly all suicide deaths is that the victim informs at least one significant individual (family member, friend, or physician) of his or her intention. Stevenson (1988) suggests that such prior information is often *disregarded by the informed person*. This tends to increase the risk of suicide.

A key method to evaluate the level of suicide ideation is to inquire about the adolescent's current suicide plan. The existence of a suicide plan is strongly associated with high risk of suicide. A plan for suicide includes: an intention to die, a method of causing harm, and preparation to carry out the plan (Hoff, 1984; Motto, 1978; Beck, Resnick, and Letteri, 1974; Robins et al., 1959; Ramsey et al., 1993).

I frequently ask adolescents with suicidal ideation, "How would you commit suicide?" Generally, the more detail in the suicide plan, the greater the level of suicidal thought. This seems to be associated with increased risk of self-harm. The next question concerning suicidal planning is whether the adolescent has access to the means necessary to carry out the plan. If a young man has a plan to shoot himself but has yet to acquire the gun, the risk is lower than if a loaded revolver is kept in the family home. Questioning the adolescent about the time line for when the suicide plan will be carried out is also important.

The individual risk factor that has received the most attention in the literature is that of previous suicide attempt history. Past behavior is often a solid predictor of future behavior, and suicide is no different in this respect. Some controversy seems to exist about what constitutes an actual suicide attempt. Does the cutting behavior of some adolescents qualify? What about adolescents who engage in high-risk behaviors such as smoking or alcohol and drug use, which can have major long term consequences?

One type of behavior that must be differentiated from suicide attempts is that of self-cutting with little suicide intent (Simpson, 1975). Clients who engage in these behaviors usually cut themselves superficially and repetitively to relieve tension precipitated by an interpersonal crisis (Brent, 1997).

Follow-up studies have shown that after one suicide attempt, the risk of violent death increases by up to three times in the six months following the initial attempt (Kaminer, Feinstein, and Barret, 1987). Estimates of the risk of repetition of suicidal behavior ranges from 10 percent upon a six-month follow up to 42 percent upon a twenty-one-month follow up, with a median reoccurrence rate of 5 to 15 percent per year (Brent et al., 1993; Cohen-Sandler, Berman, and King, 1982; Hawton and Catalan, 1987; Pfeffer et al., 1991).

As a general rule, I prefer to inquire about the circumstances of previous attempts. There is a qualitative difference between the adolescent female who overdoses, changes her mind, and tells her mother versus the adolescent who overdoses and is found by parents who have come home early from a trip. Thus, I usually ask when previous attempts occurred, reaction to the failed attempt, and family response to the previous attempt. A recent suicide attempt that features an adolescent who is angry or disappointed at still being alive is much more potent than a case in which the attempt was some time ago, the adolescent experiences regret for the attempt, and the family responds with increased vigilance and involvement.

We know from research findings that the proportion of adolescents that think about suicide (approximately 50 percent) is far greater than those that attempt it (approximately 10 percent). Physical and emotional resources provide form and meaning to a person's life and offer major protection against suicide (Litman et al., 1974;

Slater and Depue, 1981). I prefer to ask adolescents who they usually talk to when they are upset. I do not ask who they talk to when thinking about suicide, because only some adolescents have had previous experience with suicide, though all adolescents have been upset before. I am interested in whom the adolescent identifies as his or her support system. This line of questioning opens up exploration into whether the adolescent utilized the support system, and if not, how the adolescent makes sense of this decision. Another useful line of questioning is how the adolescent included some people and excluded others (perhaps family members). This provides a possible segue into the adolescent's perception of the family and larger context. It is important for the therapist not to overlook the other family members' resources (family friends), or even the resources of the community and the therapist. Generally, if adolescents have limited resources, their risk for self-harm is increased.

CONCEPTUALIZATION OF SUICIDE IN FAMILY THERAPY

How therapists conceptualize or make sense of adolescent suicidal behaviors has major repercussions for the therapeutic process. I discuss Haley's life cycle view, suicide as communication, research on common precipitating events, and present the current debate on adolescent impulsiveness and the ramifications for suicidal behaviors.

Haley (1980) suggests that all forms of nonneurological adolescent psychiatric disturbance may be viewed as an indicator of the family's failure to adjust to the psychosocially changing lifestyle of the adolescent (Wassenaar, 1987). Haley also suggests that middle to late adolescents often develop symptoms when the family does not adjust well to the launching stage of family development. An implicit assumption by Haley is that healthy development by an adolescent means developing independence from the family. Adolescents who experience difficulty in this stage are characterized as the scapegoat symptom bearers, whose families are ill-prepared for this independence.

From an interactional perspective, suicidal behavior is placed in a slightly different context. The plea character of suicidal behaviors seems to be a call for help. Why not a direct call for help? The answer may lie in the family's rules of communication, which do not permit the suicidal person to state his or her needs openly to others. The suicidal act itself is the communication that there is a problem that needs resolution (Richman, 1979).

There is a common conceptualization of suicide as manipulation. I propose that "manipulative" in this context does not describe the attribute of the adolescent but rather the caregiver relationship to the adolescent. The widespread view that suicide is manipulative lends support to my thesis that the significant relationships of the suicidal adolescent are often prevented from providing the needed support due to anxiety-producing circumstances of potential self-harm. Although caregiver reactions to threats of suicide as "manipulative" are unfortunate, it does provide the therapist an opportunity to process these responses in hopes of creating more tolerance for adolescents at risk.

The Five "Ps"

In adolescence, the five "Ps" (poverty, peers, pregnancy, parents, and punctured romance) are common events or experiences often reported as stressful precipitants to suicidal behavior. There is no clear relationship between the severity of any particular event and the emotional impact it delivers (Ramsey et al., 1993). It may help to ask adolescents about their perception of each of these events. The postmodern-influenced family therapies, such as narrative therapy, hold great promise in focusing on the coconstruction of meaning, and attempts to amplify adolescents' marginalized experiences of precipitating events.

Discord, physical and sexual abuse, exposure to family violence, and unsupportive interactions are more common in families of suicide attempters than in those of psychiatric or community controls, and also are associated with repeated suicide attempts (Furgusson and Lynskey, 1995; Kerfoot et al., 1996; Kosky, Silburn, and Zubrick, 1990; Reinhertz et al., 1995; Taylor and Stansfeld, 1984, in Brent, 1997).

I often wonder if the view of adolescents as "impulsive" prevents caregiver queries into the adolescent's lived experience of precipitating events. I think this encourages a passive stance toward the suicidal adolescent, so the adolescent may experience a disconnection from those in the position to be of most help. Impulsivity is a common characteristic of adolescent attempters. For some persons the act of suicide appears to be impulsive, occurring without planning or premeditation. These are clearly a minority group. Suicide among the young has often been assumed to be of this type. However, in actuality, the impulsive suicide attempt in response to some immediate stress is carried out by only a small number of people (Margolin and Teicher, 1968; Peck, 1985).

THERAPEUTIC PROCESS

Marriage and family therapy literature emphasizes process over content issues, although I feel that suicide presents some special struggles for the therapist. Compared to other disorders, only stomach ulcers elicit a negative, unsympathetic, unfavorable response from caregivers with a frequency remotely comparable to that for suicidal behaviors (Patel, 1975; Goldney and Bottrill, 1980).

Several studies describe caregiver responses in terms of unresponsiveness, passivity, denial, avoidance of the subject, intolerance of dependence or overprotectiveness, hostility, and a pessimistic lack of support for the patient (Wheat, 1960; Bloom, 1967; Zee, 1972; Ramon and Breyter, 1978; Birtchnell, 1983; Shneidman, 1984).

Hill (1970) found that the relatives of suicidal persons display a striking paucity of empathy, not necessarily with all persons, but with the suicidal person. Richman (1979) described family interviews which indicated that the communication between the suicidal individual and his or her family is characterized by a tendency toward the rejection of mutual communication or reciprocal give-and-take and an emphasis on secretiveness. It worries me that therapists also have difficulty showing support. I see the therapeutic process with suicidal adolescents as a juggling act between reconnecting adolescents to their support system, empowering the parents to feel they can be of help, and managing and monitoring my own reactions. Because family members' initial reactions are often negative, just involving them in therapy requires sensitivity.

I have often been asked to evaluate adolescents for discharge planning following a suicide attempt. Numerous times parents were unwilling to leave work to meet with me. Wassenaar (1987) suggests that the therapist should acknowledge all practical difficulties (work or school conflicts) but, if necessary, stress the seriousness of the adolescent's situation and offer to provide certificates and letters for employers and schools. In my experience, if a parent is unable to leave work to participate in the adolescent's therapy, it is usually less a comment on the work context of the parent than on the relationship of the parent to the suicidal adolescent. I would often indicate to reluctant parents that I thought it would be unfair of me to treat the adolescent without allowing them a voice in the process. Because caregivers may have difficulty being supportive, their attendance is a critical part of coconstructing more helpful relationships.

The general procedure in empowering parents is to join with them, empathize with their plight—the difficulties they have had and are facing—underscore their commitment as parents, and emphasize their strengths as individuals (Landau-Stanton and Stanton, 1991). Empowering parents usually requires neutralizing adolescents in some way, either by ignoring them, disparaging their thoughtlessness, or some similar means (Landau-Stanton and Stanton, 1991). This is a form of unbalancing (Minuchin, 1974).

One of the greatest risks in the treatment of suicide attempts in children and adolescents is the adoption by the therapist of moralist attitudes and consideration of the adolescent as the "victim" of the situation. The parents could be disqualified because of this posture (Vaz-Leal, 1989).

In some cases, a manipulative relapse is invoked by an outside therapist who continually centralizes the patient, exhorts the patient to share his or her true inner feelings with the therapist instead of the family, or works in some other way to undermine the parents' competencies and responsibility. It is much more important for the patient to talk honestly and revealingly to members of his or her family than to the therapist (Landau-Stanton and Stanton, 1991).

It is essential that therapy create a process that encourages more supportive relationships. I have considerable doubt as to whether this could occur if the focus privileges one part of the system while quieting the other. The influence of the reflecting team is relevant here due to the emphasis on public processes and transparency (Andersen, 1987). David Epston has introduced the term "transparency" to refer to the process of deconstructing and situating the therapist's contributions to the therapy process (Freeman and Combs, 1996).

It is certainly more valuable for the therapists to be aware of their angry or rejecting feelings than to push them away or feel self-critical for such untherapeutic attitudes. They may in fact be turned to good therapeutic use (Richman, 1979). For example, "Tim, each time you indicate that you're going to commit suicide I feel a knot in my stomach tightening and wonder how others (family members) personally react to this?"

Working exclusively with one part of the system obscures the influence of all members, and promotes a mystical quality about therapy. If a suicidal adolescent is feeling distraught and discouraged and is facing parents who are angry at not being privy to the adolescent's struggle prior to attempts on his own life, I would think that all would be keenly interested in the process of developing a reconnection to more supportive relationships. A healthy irreverence for the social utility of our own professional ideas can encourage family members to develop an irreverence for their preferred methods of handling other family members. This may help the family to self-evaluate the premises of its preferred modes of functioning, and to shift to other ways more easily.

Although to some extent all families feel discouraged and hopeless when they enter therapy, this sense of hopelessness is very pronounced in families with a suicidal adolescent. In some studies, hopelessness has been correlated with suicidal intent, suicide reattempt, and suicide completion (Beck et al., 1974; Hawton et al., 1982; Kerfoot et al., 1996). Restoration of hope even at the assessment phase is crucial to set the stage for continuing intervention (Brent, 1997).

I fondly remember an experience of interviewing Andrew, a sixteen-year-old with suicidal ideation, and his upset parents. I naively asked Andrew and his parents what they hoped for from therapy. I then received three blank looks initially, followed by a shrug of the shoulders from Andrew, and the parents replying in resignation, "We don't think anything will be a help at this point." My question was mistimed, and it became clear to me that the family needed to engage in more "problem talk" before focusing on resources and future-oriented goals. I learned from this experience that families have resources, and the therapist need not take the family's "hopeless" responses as a descriptor of the family but rather as a comment on the current therapeutic relationship.

A key concept in suicidal ideation that is often overlooked by the family therapy literature is that of ambivalence. The conflict between the wish to die and the desire to live is familiar to caregivers who intervene with suicidal persons.

Therapeutically, ambivalence is essential in helping families because it can be a vehicle to a stock of resources if timed appropriately. I recall asking Andrew and his family, "What has kept suicide out of your lives until now?" Andrew responded that he really had gotten good at fixing small appliances and electronic equipment that people had given up on, and this hobby had essentially kept him going. Andrew's mom and dad shared that before recent financial pressures, the family bickered less, ate supper together, and were more available for one another. This presented a host of possible directions to encourage supportive relationships.

How the issue of suicide is broached in therapy is of seminal importance. If the therapist seems hesitant, and/or uses vague language, the adolescent and family may conclude that the therapist is uncomfortable with the issue and its disclosure. Rating scales and psychological tests of the suicidal person and his or her significant others can be helpful, but the best way to tell if someone is suicidal is to ask the person directly in a sensitive and understanding manner (Richman, 1979).

For example, I asked Andrew after numerous red flags went up for me, "Are you thinking about killing yourself?" Andrew responded in a matter-of-fact way that he had been thinking about it for a couple of weeks. This response sometimes does not occur; thus it is important to ask the question repeatedly throughout the session.

The negative response to questions of suicidal ideation can reflect a tenuous therapeutic relationship rather than lack of suicidal thoughts. When I asked him about how he would kill himself, Andrew responded with a plan that involved carbon monoxide poisoning. I indicated to Andrew that this concerned me greatly, and I inquired into whether Andrew had access to the means necessary to carry out the plan. His parents informed me that they had a garage, and Andrew's father would often take his mother to work to save mileage on their other vehicle. Though Andrew had never attempted suicide previously, it became important to find out what resources were available to him and his family, including professional resources.

Exploration of resources beyond the boundaries of the family is often necessary in situations where relations have become chronically strained. Andrew indicated he had one close friend, Charles, who often participated in his hobby, and he found him to be "a pretty good guy." I was curious as to why Andrew did not disclose his suicidal thoughts to Charles. Andrew indicated that he did not want to burden him with it. I wondered aloud what Andrew thought Charles' reaction might be if he learned that he was not privy to Andrew's plans to kill himself.

The parents indicated that they worked full time, but Andrew's maternal grandparents were retired and lived on a nearby farm. I inquired with Andrew about his relationship with his grandparents, and he reported getting along OK but did not feel comfortable talking to them about "heavy" issues. The parents reported that the wife's parents were close to the family and had been consulted before about family struggles. I was concerned with Andrew's active suicide plan and limited resources.

A no-suicide contract is a time-limited therapeutic contract between the therapist and the at-risk adolescent. It is important to make the time frame as brief as possible because when an adolescent is actively suicidal, it is important to arrange for small successes. It is easier to agree not to harm yourself until the next day than until the next week. The contract is about not acting on suicidal thoughts but allows the adolescent to think about suicide. It is essential in the contract to identify who the adolescent will contact should he or she feel unable to keep himself or herself safe. It is important to notify identified resources about the situation and to enlist their assistance in the home safety plan. It is essential to obtain explicit agreement regarding the exclusion of suicidal behavior.

It is necessary to renegotiate the no-suicide contract at every therapeutic contact with the adolescent at risk. Coupled with the no-suicide contract is the issue of whether monitoring is required from the family or the hospital. My primary concern is for the safety of the adolescent, though a close second includes how to enhance the personal agency of all concerned regarding the risk of suicide.

The home safety watch hinges on the involvement and participation of the parents and other significant resources. It includes monitoring the adolescent twenty-four hours a day to prevent harm to the adolescent. Stanton and Stanton (1991) suggest that it is important to have a support backup for each resource person monitoring the adolescent.

I had asked Andrew's family, "How would you know that you could be reasonably sure that the home safety watch for Andrew was no longer necessary?" It is important to highlight behavioral outward indicators of progress. I think that the home safety watch can significantly enhance personal agency for the family and the adolescent.

If numerous attempts at a no-suicide contract and home safety watch fail to be established, it may be necessary to consider hospitalization. Many variations in the use of hospital resources and options provide opportunities for continued family involvement.

For some time I considered hospitalization to be counterproductive in enhancing the adolescent and family's personal agency because, essentially, the hospital staff was displacing the family's position in keeping the adolescent safe. I now think this either/or thinking was less helpful, and it was imperative that I consider ways to invite the family and adolescent to participate in the hospital stay.

> Not only do we demand parental participation before admission of an adolescent inpatient, we also require that they be *on call* for the inpatient staff whenever needed, day or night. If a problem arises with their adolescent on the unit, the parents will be called for guidance, consultation, or advice, and may be asked to come in and settle it. (Stanton and Stanton, 1991, p. 321)

Hospitalization may be indicated if there is a risk of flight, and in that case the police may be needed. Commitment procedures exist in each state as an absolute last resort should the suicidal adolescent and family be unwilling to commit to therapy, no-suicide contracts, home safety watches, or the adolescent's voluntary admission to the hospital. All options short of commitment procedures should be explored and exhausted first. Stanton and Stanton (1991) indicate that if the family is overwhelmed about implementing the home safety watch, a variation could involve placing the adolescent in the hospital over-night to give the family some respite, or have the adolescent attend a day treatment program coupled with the family's home safety watch during the reminder of the day. Hospitalization should not be implied as a failure of the adolescent or the family, but rather as another short-term resource in the process of enhancing personal agency. Inpatient admission is probably indicated if the adolescent

- has made a clearly suicidal attempt;
- makes an attempt secretively that was unlikely to be discovered;
- shows a commitment to suicide rather than just a plea for help;
- has a family history of successful suicide;
- is in a family in which members are so panic-stricken that they feel they cannot prevent the adolescent from attempting. (Stanton and Stanton, 1991)

The therapist should be firm yet empathetic and remember that the therapist should remain in charge of management decisions. The adolescents' presence in the hospital evidences their own inability to deal effectively with their situations, so they should not be allowed to prescribe their own treatment (Haley, 1980).

It should not be overlooked that family members need a means of notifying one another of future breakdowns in the family relationships that may increase the risk of suicide. This responsibility could be shared mutually between the adolescent and other family members. It may be tedious and tiresome to depend exclusively on verbal modes of inquiring about suicide, so the family may need to use some kind of nonverbal warning system. This may be accomplished by the family and adolescent agreeing on a household object that will signify "safety" or "all is well." For example, one family indicated that their safety object was a vase on the mantel. If it was missing, family members knew that someone in the family needed support. The family member who noticed the missing vase would immediately contact all family members to check to see how they were doing. This was a creative way to assess safety in family relations that may become strained.

The restoration of adolescent-family relationships is vital in keeping the suicidal adolescent safe from harm. I do not believe that family and friends are nonsupportive because they do not care. I think that living in an individualistic culture discourages reaching out to others, especially in the face of suicidal risk. The sheer terror that suicide can invoke in significant others, coupled with the tenuous nature of many of our family relationships, can create a context for the premature demise of our future generations. Therapists have the potential to be a counterforce by showcasing a therapeutic process that highlights the family's caring, compassion, and connection for one another.

SUMMARY

- Therapists need to create a context in therapy that balances the validation and acknowledgment of family members' anxiety and fears about the threat of suicide, while inviting the family to find a way to remain supportive of the adolescent's needs.
- Therapists need to monitor and manage their reactions to the threat of adolescent suicide.
- Therapists can highlight their reactions to the threat of suicide so as to invite the family members to discuss and process their reactions.
- Therapists need to access their support system of colleagues in order not to mirror the isolated nature of the suicidal adolescent.
- Therapists need to acknowledge adolescents' ambivalence about suicide.
- Therapists need to be aware of the groups of adolescents that are at increased risk for suicide.
- Suicide intent is not equated with extent of medical damage to the adolescent in previous suicide attempts.
- Always assess for suicide if the adolescent presents with depressed systems.
- Inquire repeatedly and directly about suicide. Avoid vague language that may imply that you are uncomfortable with the topic.
- Adolescent suicide attempts are rarely impulsive and usually occur with warning.

- Suicide is always an attempt to influence or communicate with others. Viewing suicide as "manipulation" blocks the therapist and the family members from being a support for the adolescent at risk.
- No-suicide contracts should be short term, be highly specified, identify resources to access, and focus on suicidal behavior, not ideation.
- Hospitalization should be used only as a last resort and the family should be invited to participate in the hospital care as much as possible.
- Families should be invited to participate in the home safety watches either in lieu of hospitalization or following discharge from the hospital.

Assessment of suicide involves:

- Details of suicide plan (plan, means, and time)
- Previous suicide behavior (individual and family history)
- Resources (adolescent's identified resources)

SECTION IV:
TREATMENT ISSUES

.

Chapter 11

Use of Self

Robert W. Marrs

Adolescence can be a real roller coaster. Decisions that might seem trivial to adults, such as what clothes to wear, what music to listen to, or what activities to get involved with, may have huge implications for adolescents and their fight for autonomy, self-confidence, and personal identity. It is also a time of constant change in physical, emotional, spiritual, and social development; changes that can bring about great excitement and joy, but great pain and frustration as well.

For adolescents presenting themselves in treatment, the therapist becomes a powerful and influential instrument of change and stability. For this reason, I believe it to be profoundly important that issues pertaining to the use of self are addressed. An adolescent will quickly see through a phony therapist or turn to stone should he or she feel a sense of distrust or insincerity. Clinicians working with families of adolescents may also find themselves confused or manipulated by the chaotic and sometimes complicated dynamics of their interaction. This chapter, therefore, is devoted to the use of self in adolescent treatment.

THE NATURAL SELF

Building relationships had always been a fairly easy process for me. People would approach me almost anywhere: on buses and planes, at work or in school, standing on a street corner, or sitting in the park. And there was always something very natural about our exchange. It was a genuine interaction among two or more people wishing to share some part of their Selves.

Then something interesting happened. I became a therapist and it all changed. I began feeling distant, anxious, and even self-conscious. It was as if professionalism—the graduate degree, the job title, and the new pair of Dockers—molded me into someone else. The natural exchanges that I had always experienced when meeting new people suddenly did not seem so natural anymore. I was afraid of failing. I was an expert, after all. I was a professional. But somehow, I was different.

Indeed, *I* was different. Not the people who came to talk to me, but I. Building the therapeutic relationship became artificial and left me somewhat removed from the client's emotional system. "Joining" was now a technique; that is, a process that once had occurred spontaneously and genuinely had become deliberate and methodological. Moreover, whenever I did enter into the client's emotional system, I became uncomfortable. My mind would quickly be filled with the various "codes of ethics" and other "do's and don'ts" that had been indoctrinated into me during my early training. I had also received the message that the more personal a therapist is, the less professional he or she can be. Maintaining that image of professionalism was very important to me as I started my career. In so doing, however, I had changed.

Fortunately, my professional development did not end there. In time, I was able to return to a more personal and intimate interaction. I credit this transformation to my clients who molded and shaped me into a more mature helper. In fact, of all the various populations and social groups I have worked with, it has been adolescents that have taught me the most. They have taught me how to love more deeply, to be more accepting and unassuming, to laugh a little louder, and to enjoy the spontaneity of life.

In my opinion, here is why: When adults present themselves for therapy, they enter taking on a professional role: the role of the client. This therapist/client relationship, however, is a socially constructed system based on either a medical model of disease and pathology, creating a doctor/patient relationship, or a postindustrial, business-oriented paradigm of professionalism—"I am the therapist and you are the client." In essence, within the context of therapy, you cannot have one without the other. This professional paradigm is not unlike that of salesperson/customer, CEO/laborer, partner/ copartner. It is a business-oriented paradigm. This paradigm, however, is not usually the best fit for therapy. It often creates a power imbalance and places a barrier in the therapeutic relationship. Each person, then, must behave according to his or her role of client or therapist. Then, because of the implications of those roles, the relationship can become preoccupied with legal-based ethics, payment arrangements, theoretical models, etc. Moreover, therapists begin to see their jobs through the lens of a "business person" instead of that of a caring helper. Therapy soon becomes a little less natural and a little more artificial.

Developmentally, adolescents are at a point in their lives when it is appropriate to challenge adults and those in authority. Adolescents simply refuse to be assigned the role of "client." For a therapist, this can become very frustrating very fast. Adolescents do not want to behave "professionally." They do not want to accommodate theoretical models, serve as lab rats for trendy interventions, or help therapists to feel professional. They simply want to "be." Therapists working with adolescents will soon find themselves at a crossroads. One can either learn to adapt one's Self to the adolescent, which means adopting a new paradigm, or throw one's hands in the air and move on to another population. Fortunately for me, I chose to adopt a new paradigm, and, in so doing, liberated my "Natural Self" from the dominant professional discourse. I soon found myself relating to my clients in a much more genuine way. Most important, the adolescents saw me as genuine and, therefore, invited me into their lives, into their "Selves."

So how does a therapist do this? How does one step out from under the old paradigm and become "more natural"? First of all, one does not "become natural." Nature is not something to be attained; it simply is what it is. We are all natural. The challenge is resisting the messages that distract us from being natural. In the therapy context, such messages might be "we shouldn't cry in front of our clients," or "we shouldn't discuss our personal lives with clients." Such messages can keep us guarded and emotionally removed. The focus tends to be more on what one "does" to the client rather than how one "is" with the client.

I believe this is due, in part, to the theory of therapy the clinician is using. For example, a therapist working from a psychoanalytic perspective is less likely to use Self interactively than someone working from a Rogerian or narrative therapy perspective. Psychoanalysis is very aware of the pitfalls that can easily occur between a client and an undifferentiated therapist, and therefore will contend that the therapist should remain outside of the system in a dispassionate way. The problem is that it creates a polarity that prohibits the relationship from being connected on a deeper level.

However, how one uses himself or herself is not just about a model of therapy. In fact, according to James Framo, "Much of what transpires between clients and therapists is expressed by tone, gestures, expression, sensory impressions, feelings, and a host of other almost incommunicable states" (Framo, 1982, p. 61). In other words, "who" the therapist is and "how" the therapist is makes all the difference in the world. From an intersubjective perspective, therapists are not immune to the interpersonal, emotional, and psychological dynamics of the therapeutic relationship. The therapist is not an observer removed from the emotional field of the therapeutic relationship, but rather an active participant with the adolescent. Therefore, the relationship tends to be mutually influential whether we are conscious of it or not (Goldenstein, 1997).

The level of comfort the therapist experiences in becoming emotionally or intimately involved with the client is also important. I contend that the therapeutic system is a relationship whereby a free exchange of Selves takes place. It is interactive in that the therapist is encouraged to participate on an intimate level with the client. This means sharing personal information, and sharing thoughts and feelings. It is a relationship not unlike those in our personal lives. That is not to say that the therapist does not act responsibly, observing the appropriate boundaries, but rather relates to the client on a deeply personal level.

Framo (1982) suggests that clients enter a therapeutic relationship with an expectation that their relationship with the therapist will be "special" or "unique"; that the therapist will give something "extra" of himself or herself. In other words, it is the expectation that the relationship will be personal and intimate.

This must be done honestly and genuinely. For example, in working with adolescents, many therapists make the mistake of trying to relate by acting like an adolescent. A teenager will see through this phony exterior and reject such a therapist as patronizing and insincere. Other therapists might be very uncomfortable sharing their Selves with adolescents for fear that they will be ridiculed in some way. After all, teenagers are masters at "pushing buttons" and exploiting weaknesses. However, the teenager will most likely interpret such a therapist as uncaring and judgmental. It has been my experience that adolescents enjoy adult role models in their lives. They need adults to be honest, forthcoming, inquisitive, and compassionate. They want to learn from the therapist and for that therapist to be genuinely "interested" in who they are as individuals: to respect their ideas, their differences, their uniqueness, and to separate their behavior from their person. Therapist self-disclosure and genuineness are significant factors in successful treatment (Anderson and Mandell, 1989, as cited in Goldenstein, 1994).

Children and adolescents have three primary needs from parents and adults (Kohut, 1971, 1977). The first is the need for a sense of positive self-worth, which is reflected in parent-teen interaction. During adolescence, teens are exploring their own "Selves," sharing ideas, creative interests, establishing a greater sense of independence. Therefore, how parents and other adults, including the therapist, react to the teen's attempts at autonomy can send powerful messages regarding that teen's sense of self-worth.

The second primary need is for a sense of stability. The many developmental changes associated with adolescence can be quite tumultuous for teens. What may seem "typical" of the adult experience may be very new for a teen and, therefore, quite frightening and anxiety producing. Teens may also have difficulty both internalizing their experiences and expressing their feelings in an emotionally mature way. Instead, the adolescent may react with intensity or project those feelings onto others. It is, therefore, important that adults react to such situations with calmness and strength: be reassuring; keep your voice low and soothing; validate, don't patronize; and be patient. Reacting in this manner will promote healthy emotional development and impart positive coping skills through the adult's own modeling behaviors.

The third primary need identified by Kohut is the need for an adult alter ego, which is able to reflect a sense of humanity and vulnerability. Again, adults—parents, teachers, therapists—play an essential role in the adolescent's development of a healthy Self. When adults show their own vulnerabilities, they model compassion and understanding. This also validates the teen's experience by showing that he or she is not abnormal and not alone. These three needs can help therapists determine how self-disclosure can be used to promote healthy development and strengthen the therapeutic bond.

One of the most powerful interventions in clinical work, especially working with adolescents, is the use of humor. Brooks (1994) suggests that humor, when used appropriately, can strengthen the therapeutic alliance and facilitate change. The use of humor teaches effective coping strategies, gives problems a sense of perspective, titrates difficult feelings, and cuts through resistance. Therapists who use humor to poke fun at themselves without being self-deprecating show great vulnerability and personal strength, a strong True Self. Furthermore, the adolescent's ability to use humor effectively may be an important factor to assess. Lack of humor or inappropriate use of humor may provide important information regarding how the adolescent views himself or herself and the world.

I spent a number of years facilitating adolescent therapy groups. My approach was simply to be myself—to be a responsible adult in charge of maintaining the hierarchy and structure of the group and to do so through the sharing of my successes as well as my failures. David Keith and Carl Whitaker (1987) remind us that failure is a natural part of life, even for therapists. Our failures build character and, oftentimes, open new doors of opportunity and growth. We should share our past experiences of failure with our clients, especially adolescents. By being open and vulnerable, we share in the emotional experience of adolescents and help them to see that failures are normal, expected, and temporary.

Keith and Whitaker (1987) also suggest that failure in therapy is more likely to occur when we cease to be natural by either losing ourselves in our professionalism or allowing our own "problems" to emerge in self-serving, self-gratifying ways. We are not the "all-knowing, all-powerful, all-loving" experts that we may think we are. We are fallible human beings who make mistakes and do not always have the answers.

Eda Goldenstein (1994) suggests that self-disclosure must be done with an attunement to the adolescent's needs and relationship history, which calls for an understanding and awareness of the metarelationship between the adolescent and the therapist. Depending on those needs, there may be circumstances when therapist self-disclosure is intrusive or reflective of hurtful relationships in the adolescent's life. For example, oftentimes children and adolescents are triangulated into the role of confidant with adults. This can result in inappropriate expectations and call for the child or adolescent to assume an emotional responsibility that is beyond the bounds of a healthy relationship or beyond his or her developmental capacity. Self-disclosure in this case could create an unhealthy and harmful isomorph of past relationships.

Self-disclosure can also be problematic for adolescents who show signs of poor reality testing or who struggle to maintain appropriate boundaries. Depending on the client's diagnosis or relationship history, self-disclosure may be experienced as too intimate and threatening and clients may misinterpret the intentions of the therapist. Other clients may use self-disclosure to avoid facing difficulties (Goldenstein, 1994). Ultimately, self-disclosure should be used to enhance the therapeutic relationship while protecting the adolescent client from potential harm.

Finally, clinicians may need to process personally revealed information with the adolescent. In other words, process the meaning the adolescent has given to the information being shared (Stolorow, Brandchaft, and Atwood, 1994, as cited in Goldenstein, 1997). Does the adolescent understand clearly and accurately what is being shared? What meaning has he or she given to the shared information? How is the information helpful to the adolescent's situation or to the therapeutic relationship? Processing personal information can lead to a greater appreciation and understanding of the adolescent's subjective world, providing new directions for treatment.

Keith and Whitaker (1987) remind us that sometimes what we as therapists believe is ineffectual or a failure in therapy, might actually produce positive change in the client or family. It was in my experience of personal failure that I learned one of the most important lessons in adolescent treatment. I had been relating very well with an adolescent, but had not felt as though I was effective in my interventions or even clear in my sense of direction. Yet the adolescent was becoming more and more open with me as we continued to spend time together. In experiencing this situation with a number of other adolescents, I realized that it was my relationship, and the attributes of that relationship, that was influencing positive change.

Conversely, adolescents and families may also interpret the therapeutic process or their own efforts as a failure when they are, in fact, not failures at all. For example, as parents begin to implement appropriate structure with an oppositional child or adolescent, there might initially be an increase in acting-out behaviors as the child or adolescent attempts to test the parents' resolve. Oftentimes, parents will become frustrated, interpreting this increase in opposition as a failure in their parenting and, consequently, project a sense of hopelessness onto the child or adolescent. My role as a therapist is to help parents understand that this increase in opposition is a normal stage in the change process. In other words, things could get worse before they get better.

Being myself with adolescents also meant respecting their ideas whether I agreed with those ideas or not. It meant caring for them whether they were behaving appropriately or not. And it meant laughing and having a good time. In this way, I was able to create a context for change. Usually after the first few days in the group, an adolescent would drop his or her tough facade and become more open and genuine. A sense of safety and trust would be established between us and among the teens themselves. Furthermore, the relationship that developed with the teen would be in and of itself a powerful model for the family. But the key was that the relationship was interactive, which allowed me to be invited into the relationship system.

One afternoon, just before my adolescent group was to start, I heard the outside doorbell ring. Standing outside was one of my adolescent clients and two other teens that I had never met. My client had gone home and encouraged two of her friends to come and be a part of the group. She had told them that she was getting a lot out of the group and they might benefit from it as well. This was a very powerful statement to me about the bond that this teen had built with me as well as the cohesion of the group. Curious about this, I pulled the teen aside to ask her why the group was so important to her that she would want to invite her friends. She said, "Because you look out for us, and it's fun."

A therapist who is interactive with his or her clients opens the door for something wonderful to happen. It opens the door for personal growth. I believe that each and every client can contribute something positive and meaningful to our lives. They can teach us about ourselves, about their own lives and the lives of their families, and about the world around us. They teach us to be better therapists, better brothers or sisters, better parents, or better spouses. But a therapist must give himself or herself permission to learn. The therapist must have a strong True Self and be vulnerable. If we do so, the therapeutic relationship will be a transformative process for the client as well as the therapist.

THE FIGHT FOR CONTROL

Probably most therapists working with adolescents are doing so in a group therapy situation, whether it is inpatient, partial hospital, or intensive outpatient treatment. Working with an adolescent on a one-to-one basis is one thing, but working with an entire group of adolescents can be quite another matter. If therapists struggle in this environment, it is usually due to one thing: the fight for control. Adolescents can be impulsive, unpredictable, and oftentimes hot-headed. Even a veteran therapist can lose his or her sense of control over the situation very quickly.

In my experience, one of two things may happen. The therapist's reactivity to adolescent group behaviors will either cause that therapist to become overly authoritarian—becoming too quick to discipline, establishing unreasonable goals, showing intolerance of otherwise normal adolescent behaviors, losing effective nurturing behaviors, becoming physically and verbally aggressive—or, contrariwise, the therapist can become overly permissive—allowing negative behaviors to go unchallenged. In either case, the structure of the group will rapidly deteriorate and staff will spend most of their time "putting out fires" instead of conducting effective therapy.

The notion of countertransference—the therapist's own reactivity to the client—is important to consider when working with adolescents. Proctor (1959) points out that adolescents who are physically and verbally aggressive, impulsive, narcissistic, and/or oppositional are most likely to elicit countertransference or counterreaction problems. Such counterreactions may include counterattacking, and/or punitive or authoritarian responses. The therapist can also be pulled into the position of defending himself or herself to the adolescent. This will quickly undermine therapist credibility. Furthermore, it is important to be mindful that such counterreactions may, in fact, be isomorphic of other adult-child or parent-child interactions in the teen's life. Mishne (1996, p. 141), therefore, encourages clinicians to seek consultation, supervision, and psychotherapy regularly. This allows therapists to prevent such counterreactions from occurring by increasing self-awareness, learning effective management strategies, and promoting greater differentiation, which will be discussed in the next section.

An appropriate group structure is one in which the therapist establishes an authoritative environment. It is an equal balance of positive behavior management and emotional nurturing. The therapist is able to remain appropriately dispassionate to negative behavior and compassionate to emotional needs. Positive behavior management means that rules and consequences are issued fairly and consistently. Adolescents need to know that there is a sense of justice and fair play in the group. The alternative is an impression of favoritism or personal bias, which will increase the likelihood of negative behaviors. Emotional nurturing means the therapist sees past negative behaviors to the true heart of the individual. Judgment is reserved for the clients until you have taken the time to really get to know them and the story they have to tell. Most important, remind them constantly of their strengths, talents, and achievements. In a healthy, structured environment such as this, adolescents will begin to feel safe and cared for. Only then will a therapist be able to address the deeper issues that brought them into treatment.

THE DIFFERENTIATED THERAPIST

Edwin Friedman (1991), in his writing on Bowenian theory, defines differentiation as "a lifelong process that is achieved through reciprocal external and internal processes of self-definition and self-regulation" (p. 140). It is an intrapsychic process that allows one to transcend to a level of objectivity and clarity regarding a relationship or an experience. This does not mean a "cutting off" of emotion, but rather an integration of one's emotive and reasoning processes. It is a process that allows therapists to maintain their sense of self despite whatever experiences they are faced with; it is maintaining the "I" within the "we."

In family systems that lack the appropriate boundaries necessary to maintain a well-functioning homeostatic structure, a loss of one's True Self can occur due to possible shifting alliances, triangles, and projections. Instead, a Pseudo Self (Bowen, 1985) emerges that is defined by the volatility of the relationship system and, therefore, greatly influenced by emotion. This Pseudo Self is a fluid, constantly shifting self that borrows not only principles and beliefs of others, but also tends to see itself *through* the eyes of others. An individual with a strong Pseudo Self and a weak True Self will struggle to maintain his or her sense of "I" within the "we." In other words, the individual is not clearly defined and, therefore, runs the risk of entering relationships that can either lead to enmeshment or polarity (Bowen, 1985).

> A thirty-five-year-old woman presented herself for therapy soon after she had broken up with her boyfriend of two years. She was depressed, confused, and frightened. In exploring her relationship history, it was revealed that she would enter into one relationship after the next with little or no time in between. Her relationships would be rather intense and last only a short time. This pattern began in early adolescence and continued to the present.

This type of pattern suggests a strong Pseudo Self in which the young woman tends to define herself solely by her relationships and, therefore, experiences great fear and confusion when single and on her own. This client will risk repeating the same relationship patterns over and over due to an inability to separate or differentiate from the relationship experience. Being unable to process a relationship or event with objectivity and clarity makes it difficult for one to learn and grow from the process, thereby strengthening the True Self.

Differentiation first becomes essential with families. In fact, the family is probably the most powerful and influential social system there is. Differentiation, therefore, allows people the ability to navigate and negotiate these powerful family forces in a way that gives us the best chance for happiness and self-fulfillment. The therapeutic process should promote differentiation.

However, if therapists have not successfully individuated from their own families of origin, resolved old relationships, or learned from past experiences, they run the same risk of being undifferentiated and, therefore, developing a Pseudo Self. From a cybernetic perspective, this has profound implications. In fact, Bowen (1985) would contend that the client is unable to progress past the maturity of the therapist. He believes that the therapist with a strong Pseudo Self, or who has not successfully differentiated from past relationship experiences, will stunt the growth of the client and, in some cases, may even do harm.

One reason for this is that a person with a low level of differentiation will tend to enmesh or polarize himself or herself in an emotional system, especially a strong emotional system. If an undifferentiated therapist is pulled into the system, he or she will most likely be tossed about like a ship on the ocean, becoming caught up in the chaotic relationship dynamics or triangulated. On the other hand, the therapist may tend toward polarity, which leaves him or her detached from the client. This affects the therapist's ability to join and empathize with the client, which may inhibit the client from progressing in therapy, create resistance, or lead the client to drop out altogether.

In working with adolescent clients and their families, clarity, objectivity, and multipartiality are especially important. Most often the adolescent is presented for therapy as the identified patient by the parents. Immediately, this creates a plaintiff-versus-defendant duality that is further accentuated by the difference in hierarchy. An undifferentiated therapist working with such a family may be inclined to take sides with either the adolescent or with the parents. The therapist, therefore, may find himself or herself being pulled from different directions and triangulated into different relationships. The therapeutic relationship or context can quickly become an isomorph of the family system.

Cybernetic theory (Bateson, 1972, 1979) also reminds us that how therapists interpret the relationship system they are working with depends greatly on their own epistemology: past experiences, relationships, values, and beliefs. One's epistemology leads one to ask certain questions, choose certain models or theories, assess relationships in a particular way, and it also influences which interventions one uses. An undifferentiated therapist runs the risk of making faulty and even irrational interpretations regarding the relationship system he or she is working with. It almost results in a sort of "tunnel vision" that prohibits the therapist from seeing the bigger picture in an objective way. An example of this occurred when I was working in a chemical dependency treatment program. It was typical that the majority of counselors in that field were former alcoholics and drug addicts. It was my observation that sometimes counselors would diagnose dependency where there was not sufficient evidence, or they would oversimplify the client's use as the primary problem and, therefore, scapegoat the identified patient. It could be argued that such counselors had not effectively differentiated from their own past substance dependency history, which led to a distorted view of family functioning.

The period of adolescence by nature is a time of differentiating. Teenagers are becoming aware of the outside world. They are testing time-honored family beliefs and traditions against what they learn from others in school, through personal experiences, and in the media. They struggle to integrate these new experiences and ideas into their own schema in a clear and objective way. This is also true for the family of a teenager. Only through clarity and objectivity will the family be able to reorganize itself in such a way that the teen can individuate and develop a stronger True Self, while preserving positive relationships among family members. For such a family presenting in therapy, the differentiated therapist can be a powerful instrument to help the family do just that.

THE USE OF SELF AND STAGES OF THERAPY

The phenomenon of therapy can be quite complex. Personalities, epistemologies, contexts, interventions, theories, and the like all contribute in different ways to make up the therapeutic milieu. Nevertheless, therapy tends to follow a specific course. James Alexander (1988) posits that therapy is a process that involves specific phases or stages from intake to termination and that these phases are common among most therapeutic contexts despite theoretical model or treatment modality. These phases are the introduction/joining phase, the assessment/understanding phase, the induction/motivation phase, the behavior/change phase, and the termination phase.

A therapist's use of self can be somewhat different at each of these phases of therapy. How I relate to an adolescent or family at intake is likely to be different than how I present myself at later phases in the process. In the following section, I will discuss each of these specific phases and how I tend to use self accordingly.

Introduction/Joining Phase

The introduction/joining phase is the initial stage in the therapeutic process. It is the time when clinicians attempt to build a sense of rapport and credibility. This can be a crucial stage for successful adolescent treatment. Joining with adolescents tends to take more time than joining with other age groups. Oftentimes adolescents will present with a sort of "tough guy" or "tough girl" exterior. They may come across as arrogant, aloof, disconcerting, oppositional, ridiculing, etc. They will often try to send a message that they are in charge and that any successful therapy that occurs is because they allow it to happen. The fight for control happens immediately.

In my experience, a therapist will make a crucial error if he or she tries to force the issue. The therapist should be sure to enforce group rules and structure, but be careful not to react to the adolescent's attitude. Rather, the therapist is better off giving the adolescent permission to be "tough." In other words, instead of engaging in a tug-of-war, simply let go of the rope. Go with the resistance, not against it. Here's why: During the initial phase of therapy, adolescents are very self-protective. In a group of peers, the tough exterior helps the adolescent hide vulnerabilities and negotiate how best to relate to peers. This allows the adolescent to achieve a sense of acceptance. An adolescent will not open up or comply with treatment in the group setting unless he or she feels a sense of belonging. Group cohesion is essential. Therefore, if a therapist reacts to the adolescent by trying to strip him or her of that tough exterior, the therapist may run the risk of exploiting the adolescent and creating a barrier to group cohesion. In an involuntary program, this could result in increased acting-out behaviors. In a voluntary group, one may simply lose the adolescent altogether.

In an individual therapy context, the adolescent may use this tough exterior to test the adult therapist. It is important to remember that underneath that attitude is likely a soft, sensitive, hurting person who longs for connection and understanding. Adolscents will not begin to reveal that side unless they feel a sense of trust, genuine appreciation, and acceptance from the adult therapist. Again, the tough exterior allows the adolescent to protect himself or herself until it is otherwise safe.

Furthermore, if an adolescent is involved in therapy, one can assume part of the problem is a loss of control or perceived loss of control over his or her life. This may be the result of a chaotic, abusive, or distant family structure or the adolescent's feelings of being out of control. It is important, therefore, to allow the adolescent the opportunity to negotiate the therapeutic relationship. If a therapist reacts to the resistance and attempts to force the adolescent to follow his or her own agenda, it may reify the adolescent's own sense of powerlessness and hopelessness.

Establishing credibility is different with an adolescent than with an adult. Adolescents typically are not concerned with titles or degrees. What seems to be more important is how well one interacts with them. They tend to care more about whether or not the therapist is someone who will keep them safe and whether or not the therapist is going to be someone they can talk to.

When Josh started his first day in the adolescent program, he strutted through the door wearing baggy pants, a backward cap, metal chains, and talking as if he owned the neighborhood. He was quick to criticize the program as well as me.

However, I could tell he was self-conscious and worried about making a good impression with his peers. This was a different side of Josh, who had presented himself as rather docile and subdued just twenty minutes earlier during his intake. Understanding that Josh was probably feeling somewhat nervous, I purposely avoided any conversations regarding his appearance. I also avoided commenting on Josh's language unless it was derogatory or excessively vulgar. Instead, I clarified group expectations and gave gentle cues when behavior became inappropriate. I was just going to let Josh be Josh so long as it did not disrupt the structure of the group. This was an important move in that it sent a message to both Josh and the group at large that I was neither intimidated nor frustrated with his attitude. Instead, it sent a message of acceptance and control. Josh's antics continued for about four days and then gradually began to disappear.

Julie was a fourteen-year-old adolescent female who presented in very much the same way. She was dressed in a Gothic style with white makeup, black lipstick and fingernail polish, and purple-dyed hair. She was a sight to behold. Julie had been referred to me for individual therapy by the local middle school. She had established quite a history of detentions and absences. There was also some concern that Julie might have been using illicit drugs because of her rebellious and oppositional behaviors. I could tell just from our introduction that she was not going to cooperate too easily with me either. Therefore, the joining and assessment phases of our work together centered on learning more about who Julie was as a person and how she thought about the world. I did not ask any questions about her family or her problems until later in the process. And I never, ever asked or commented about her apparel. By the fourth session, Julie was talking openly about her family and the events that brought her into therapy. We continued to do very good work together. Things might have gone differently had I overtly reacted to her resistance.

My approach is to allow the adolescent to be tough within the confines of an appropriate structure. I am clear regarding group rules and expectations, yet I allow for flexibility. I keep the context open for creative expression and exploration. I recognize that any conversation can have therapeutic value. I make an effort to identify attributes about each adolescent that I genuinely appreciate and enjoy. I am firm, but calm. I try to be uplifting. And I have fun.

Assessment/Understanding Phase

During both the introduction and assessment phases of treatment, it is important for therapists to take the time to effectively and thoughtfully prepare the adolescent and his or her family for the process of therapy (Mishne, 1996). Informed consent not only involves discussion regarding rules, payment arrangements, legal and ethical guidelines, and the like, but also takes away the mystery of therapy. Clinicians should foreshadow what will likely take place over the duration of treatment and what possible side effects or outcomes could occur. It may also be important to educate the adolescent and his or her family regarding the continuum of care and where the client is on the continuum. This will increase the likelihood of family involvement and strengthen the therapeutic alliance.

This phase also involves a multidimensional assessment of the adolescent's world. To make an accurate assessment, a therapist must interview people from as many contexts of functioning as possible. This includes school personnel, family members, peer groups, physicians, department of human service workers, juvenile probation officers, and employers. This will help the clinician know more about the adolescent's strengths and liabilities. For example, who shares alarm or concern in the presenting problem, which person or persons will need to be included in the therapy process in order to promote change, and what treatment model will best match the adolescent given his or her developmental readiness (Mishne, 1996).

In my experience, adolescents are more likely to tell the truth regarding others, and less likely to tell the truth regarding themselves. That is, the teen will likely be honest about people or situations in his or her life that are causing harm, especially problems in the family. However, the teen will be less likely to share information that will incriminate himself or herself, such as skipping class, substance use, etc. Therefore, it is important to involve people from other systems to gather important information and to piece together the clearest possible picture of the problem. I will also remind myself that by being vulnerable, honest, and forthcoming, I will be more likely to invite vulnerability and openness from the adolescent.

> Laura was having a lot of problems at school. She was not turning in homework nor was she attending a full week of classes. Also, she would have outbursts of anger whenever teachers or other students would confront her. Her parents were very upset and the school was running out of ideas. I decided to arrange a meeting between school personnel, the family, and my treatment team. With all parties involved talking openly about the situation, some interesting pieces of information were revealed. First, Laura's parents were divorced and living in separate places. However, because of her problems at school, both parents had become so involved in parenting her that neither one felt free to pursue new relationships. Also, the school was trying to diffuse Laura's behavior by allowing her to go to the guidance office whenever she was feeling "out of control." Basically, she was manipulating the situation. This manipulation was creating a barrier to Laura's own ability to heal from the divorce. The school began setting stronger boundaries that kept Laura in class. The family decided to set stronger boundaries as well but also increased the amount of time the family spent together talking and having fun. This allowed Laura the opportunity to confront her feelings about the divorce.

Induction/Motivation Phase

James Alexander (1988) describes the induction/motivation phase as creating a climate for change. It includes using such skills as reframing, relabeling, and validation. It includes creating a positive and hopeful environment as well as a trusting relationship. This phase of therapy overlaps the previous phases in that building a therapeutic relationship and establishing a safe context is an ongoing process. An example of this might be an adolescent or family that has already been involved in the social service system and may have a sense of distrust or fear of judgment from professionals.

Validating past negative experiences and highlighting strengths is, therefore, crucial from the beginning.

It is important to note that informed consent, discussed in the previous section, is also an ongoing process. Clinicians should be mindful that clients, especially adolescent clients, are not as expert as they are regarding psychotherapy and, therefore, may need to be reminded throughout the treatment process of what to expect. For example, I once worked with a young adolescent female who was quite resistant and closed off during the initial phase of treatment. As I began to join with her, she gradually became more and more open and honest regarding problems in her life. I had a sense of possible sexual abuse, and as I began to feel her growing sense of trust and willingness to share that knowledge, I felt it important to remind her that I was a mandatory reporter and what that would entail should she reveal such information. In this way trust was maintained, further strengthening the therapeutic alliance.

Creating a climate for change means not only validating the seriousness of the situation, but also looking for the humor in it as well. A great way to introduce humor is to poke a little fun at yourself. Adolescents seem to thrive on humor and playfulness. They enjoy lighthearted bantering and opportunities to be silly. When therapists allow themselves to be a little silly, it helps take away some of the stiffness of that business-oriented professionalism discussed earlier.

Behavior/Change Phase

Specific interventions are most likely going to be implemented in the behavior/change phase. By this time, the therapist has a working hypothesis of the problem and framework to maneuver from. Assumedly, this framework will incorporate the adolescent's frame of reference and personal identity. One also needs to account for the developmental stage of each adolescent as well as unique personality characteristics, all of which may influence the theoretical model one chooses to work from. Working with adolescents can make for some interesting challenges with regard to theoretical model and specific interventions. Therapists should, nevertheless, work from a framework that allows them to remain genuine and true to Self.

Termination Phase

Alexander (1988) points out that terminating therapy can be a difficult experience for both client and therapist. Therefore, therapists need to be very sensitive to how they manage this final phase of the process. This is especially true with adolescents.

I discovered quickly that although I had officially terminated with an adolescent—discharge summaries were typed, aftercare plans were made, and satisfaction questionnaires were filled out—the adolescent kept showing up and making contact. For an adolescent, the therapeutic relationship can have tremendous meaning and value. It may be that the therapist has been one of the teen's best or even only resources of hope, encouragement, strength, understanding, and safety. So, for a time, the adolescent may need to keep regular contact. Therapists need to understand that this is both normal and helpful in adolescent treatment. Too many times I have seen helping professionals try to enforce rigid boundaries and even label the adolescent as "dependent." Adolescents will terminate contact when they feel confident that other areas of their life are going well, but it needs to be in their time.

> George was a seventeen-year-old adolescent that I worked with for about five months in a day treatment program. We had worked very well together and genuinely enjoyed our sessions together. The first few months after treatment had been terminated, I continued to receive regular phone calls from him. He would share successes and process failures. He would ask questions and want opinions. He wanted to know he was going to be all right and to keep working at things. Although the frequency of calls diminished over time, we remained in contact for approximately two years after termination of treatment. George has since graduated from college and is a confident, responsible young man.

In some respects, this is not unlike a younger child who, while exploring a new environment, will occasionally run back to his or her parent and grab a hand or a leg. The child needs to have the security of knowing that the parent is present and accessible in order to venture out. Adolescents need the same security. Although they are eager to become adults responsible for their lives, it is still important to know that a caring, competent adult is accessible if needed. Terminating, therefore, is not necessarily complete in a single session. It may require a period of "weaning" that can take weeks, even months.

SUMMARY

Bowen suggested that differentiating was a lifelong process (Friedman, 1991). If that is true, and I believe it is, then I think it speaks to the importance of ongoing supervision in therapy. Supervision helps the therapist to remain objective and clear about the work that he or she is doing. Framo (1982) suggests that supervision must allow for personal development beyond the realm of technique and model. "It is the personal development of trainees which will determine their effectiveness as family therapists in dealing with the 'gut' issues of family life—the passions, hates, loves, injustices, sacrifices, comforts, disappointments, frustrations, ambivalences, and gratifications of family life" (p. 224). Supervision gives therapists a venue in which to do just that. By receiving important feedback from colleagues, therapists gain insight into the many ways they punctuate the interactions they have with their clients. This will help therapists work through their own personal biases and prejudices about such things as gender, culture, ethnicity, etc., as well as past experiences, all of which can prevent them from properly differentiating, and therefore working with clients to the best of their abilities. In essence, it allows therapists to reflect, integrate, adapt, and develop their epistemologies. The $64,000 question is: are therapists willing to be that vulnerable? If not, is it fair for them to expect the same from their clients? Are therapists willing to let the adolescents they treat teach and mold them? If so, therapists will enjoy the magical journey that lies ahead of them.

Chapter 12

Some Considerations on Inviting the Participation of Adolescents in Psychotherapy

Darren A. Wozny

A common emphasis in adolescent mental health programming and psychotherapy is the psychoeducational focus on correcting skill deficits. This approach might dominate the field because adolescents are seen as having less life experience than helping professionals, so there might be a tendency to presume that adolescents lack skills. A different approach is taken in this chapter. The enhancement of adolescent personal agency while balancing concerns of accountability, cognitive development, parental interests, and ethics are discussed. Harnessing adolescents' creativity, strengths, resources, and ideas is a tall order for psychotherapists, especially when faced with problems that seem to sideswipe adolescents' preferred paths of living.

FROM THE OUTSIDE LOOKING IN

In recent years, marriage and family therapists have become sensitive to issues of oppression of marginalized discourses relating to gender, race, class, and sexual orientation. For example, Rachel Hare-Mustin (1987) suggested that traditional family therapy neglected the issue of power differences between women and men. Adolescents may experience a similar form of marginalization (Stacey and Lopston, 1995). Stacey and Lopston (1995) suggested that adolescents are in a malleable stage of development compared to adults, so therapists should exercise caution regarding their influence in shaping children's lives and narratives.

Adolescents enter therapy often at the nudge of their parents, and there is the inherent danger of assuming they are not "customers" for therapy. Berg and Miller (1992) talk of "hidden customers" that could not have been identified from the presenting problem and certainly would have been missed if the therapist prematurely elected to banish the adolescent to the waiting room in favor of working with the parents. As a general rule, I like to inquire about the adolescent's view regarding the parents' decision to attend therapy and how comfortable the adolescent would be with being "cut out of the loop" should the youth decide not to return. Berg and Miller (1992) describe various therapist-client relationships, and adolescents often are assumed to enter therapy as "visitors," present only at the request of a parent or other authority figure. It should not be forgotten that these types of therapist-client relationships are not static and can change in the course of therapy.

"In conjoint sessions with adolescents and his parents, the teenager often becomes belligerent or refuses to say anything. These are such common occurrences that, as a general rule, we rarely meet conjointly with family members who are in significant conflict with each other. The therapist's maneuverability is made greater if he meets with them separately" (Fisch, Weakland, and Segal, 1982, p. 37).

Although separate interviews might be warranted in highly volatile situations, the "divide and conquer" stance of the Mental Research Institute's (MRI) approach may affect the personal agency of both the adolescent and his or her parents. The next time a volatile situation arises in their relationship, it may be problematic that the family has learned to approach one another as opponents in a life struggle of dueling agendas.

The passive role of adolescents in health care may be a contributing factor in the acquisition of "poor" health habits (Igoe, 1991). Igoe's (1991) interest is health promotion, and her concern is how children and adolescents are systematically excluded from taking an active role in their own health care. The goal of finding ways to invite adolescents to be active participants in their own wellness involves therapists as much as doctors.

Tom Andersen's (1992) work on reflecting teams has influenced my ideas regarding working with adolescents because he broadened the view of professional practice away from "private talk" toward more open dialogue. "Who of you particularly liked the idea of coming to therapy and who were more wary about it?" (Andersen, 1992). The very process of answering this question permits adolescents to have a voice in the therapy. Andersen (1992) also reports that he has gotten into the habit of asking clients, "If you really were not comfortable with this therapy, how would I know this?" I like the question because it is at a process level and discusses the relationship between the client system and the therapist system. The question discusses a method that the client system could use to alert the therapist system that the process is off track.

For example, after numerous attempts to engage a new adolescent client named Michael, and after being repeatedly greeted with a plethora of "I don't knows" and shoulder shrugs coupled with his parents' expectant looks, I decided to verbalize the anxiety concerning my temptation to excuse Michael from therapy. This permitted me to share with Michael that part of me understood it was not his idea to attend therapy and he therefore should not be forced to participate against his will, though the other part of me felt it was horribly unfair for Michael to sit in the waiting room while I discussed with his parents an issue that certainly concerned him. With the dilemma now "public" for the family, Michael could make an informed decision on whether to participate at that time.

Though family therapists often exclude children and adolescents from therapy in favor of working with parents, there is also the danger of preferring to work solely with the adolescent and dismissing the family.

Not knowing refers to the attitude and belief that the therapist does not have access to privileged information, can never fully understand another person, and always needs to learn more about what is said or known (Anderson, 1995). The not-knowing stance is a basic necessary step to creating room for adolescents to share their "lived experience," though therapists need to self-evaluate whether their questions are vehicles or roadblocks to participation.

RESEARCH IN SUPPORT OF INCREASED
ADOLESCENT INVOLVEMENT
IN THE FAMILY PROCESS

A growing body of research suggests that adolescents from families that encourage "personal agency" fare better than their counterparts. Baumrind (1978) proposed four parenting types based on levels of parental responsiveness and parental demandingness. Parental responsiveness refers to the degree to which parents respond to the child's needs in an accepting, supportive manner (Steinberg, 1999). Parental demandingness refers to the extent to which the parent expects and demands mature, responsible behavior from the child (Steinberg, 1999). Authoritative parenting reflects high levels of both parental responsiveness and demandingness; authoritarian parenting reflects lower levels of parental responsiveness and high parental demandingness; indulgent parenting refers to high levels of parental responsiveness and lower levels of parental demandingness; and indifferent parenting refers to lower levels of both parental responsiveness and demandingness (Maccoby and Martin, 1983).

Johnson, Shulman, and Collins (1991) found that perceptions of incongruent parenting were most frequent among adolescents lowest in self-esteem. They also found that the frequency of authoritative congruent parenting decreased linearly from the fifth to eighth to eleventh grades, whereas the frequency of incongruent parenting/ father authoritarian increased as a linear function of grade (Johnson, Shulman, and Collins, 1991). This suggests adolescents tend to struggle in families where the parental view of "my way or the highway" dominates.

Smetana's (1995) research with adolescents and their families suggests that families need to adapt to changing jurisdictions:

> Conflict forces parents to re-evaluate the limits of their authority and the boundaries of adolescents' personal jurisdiction. As parents appeal to social convention, the adolescent rejects their parent's perspective, and the adolescent's reinterpretation of conventions as legitimately under their personal jurisdiction form a continual dialectic in which the boundaries of parental authority are subtly transformed. (pp. 32-33)

Mounts and Steinberg (1995) found that among adolescents in low to moderate authoritative homes, higher peer drug use was related to higher use in the participants, while for adolescents in highly authoritative homes, the link did not hold. Steinberg and colleagues (1992) also found the correlation between parental involvement and adolescents' academic performance varied as a function of the level of parental authoritativeness, such that the link was stronger in more highly authoritative homes. All of these studies suggest that adolescents thrive in a context where caregivers acknowledge and attempt to address the changing needs of the adolescents while holding the youth accountable for their age-appropriate responsibilities. The isomorphism between the context of authoritative parenting and therapeutic approaches that emphasize the collaborative relationship of therapist-adolescent-family should not be missed. If therapists experience "knee-jerk" reactions to adolescents' sometimes high-risk behavior, there is a danger of falling into the quagmire of the authoritarian parents, who often invite a symmetrical power struggle with the adolescent over jurisdiction or accountability.

ACCOUNTABILITY

Accountability refers to being responsible for the effects and implications of one's actions to both oneself and those to whom one relates. Combrinck-Graham (1989) suggested children who are diagnosed as having an emotional disturbance or mental illness are viewed as being not accountable for their actions. Diagnostic systems were developed to allow psychiatrists to have a common language and to facilitate better communication, though labels do carry the baggage of "if I'm sick, I am not responsible." This kind of thinking can paralyze a therapist because if the family and adolescent believe the adolescent is "sick," all one can do is let the illness run its course and hope for a good outcome. This suggests that if dichotomous categories are used, one can invite families to redefine their problem in order to promote more hopefulness and personal agency. In my experience, families seem reluctant to abandon their diagnoses.

Given this reluctance, how can therapists integrate diagnoses in a way that promotes accountability? I posed a similar question to a workshop presenter who suggested that clients can still maintain personal agency. For example, she indicated that if an adolescent is on medication for depression, she inquires as to what percentage of the progress to date can be attributed to the medication and what percentage to the adolescent. This invites clients to take a more active role in their well-being.

Adolescence is a time when children are expected to accept more responsibility, but they may be subtly excused from accepting responsibility if

- diagnoses are used as the primary explanation for a problem;
- we insist their peers are a negative influence;
- we assume they did not fully understand what was expected of them; or
- we view the adolescent as a helpless victim of genetics and/or family history.

I often like to ask adolescents who are complaining about their parents' expectations regarding curfews and calling home, "What does it mean to you that your parents are shifting a lot of responsibility to you and have the full expectation that you can handle it?"

Parent Accountability

Accountability is not strictly the domain of the adolescent. When children fail to mend their ways in the face of extraordinary measures, it is more likely that there is an issue of "parent believability" than of child incorrigibility (Combrinck-Graham, 1989). Parental accountability is a crucial piece of working with adolescents because although very often the parents' attempts at limit setting are reasonable and viable, if there is a history of inconsistent parent-adolescent relationship, the adolescent may not quite be ready to forgive Mom and Dad. I worked with an adolescent girl and her parents. The parents had had prolonged periods of substance abuse, but were no longer abusing substances, and were experiencing trouble implementing their reasonable ideas for putting more structure into their daughter's life. The daughter was still very angry and hurt that they "were not there" for her, and she needed an opportunity to validate her experiences and hold her parents accountable before she would cooperate with their new consistent parenting efforts.

Therapist Accountability

The therapist is accountable for activating the healing resources within the family, and the family (including the adolescent) is accountable for acting upon those resources for their own healing (Combrinck-Graham, 1989). This implies that the therapist is responsible for cocreating a context for change, and the clients are responsible for taking advantage of it. The therapist who is truly accountable recognizes the limits of his or her role and responsibility in order not to contribute to the incompetence of the family system (Combrinck-Graham, 1989).

I had the preconceived notion that holding an adolescent accountable would inevitably invite a power struggle isomorphic to the struggle in the family, interfere with the therapeutic relationship, and not relate to my attempt to empower the adolescent to solve his or her problems. For the youngsters, this failure to be held accountable actually leads to a greater sense of anomie, powerlessness, and lack of control because their behavior is not taken seriously or personally; they begin to lose their sense of personal influence (Combrinck-Graham, 1989).

During my supervision experiences, a common euphemism from the supervisor was, "You are working harder than the client." Initially, I naively thought it was good that my supervisor thought I was working hard, which I was. Further consideration made me conclude that it was my supervisor's indirect way of telling me that I was interfering with the clients' personal agency.

"Self-agency: the ability to act, feel, and think in a way that is liberating, that opens up new possibilities or simply allows us to see that new possibilities exist. When I think of the word self-agency, I think of the *f* word: freedom" (Anderson, 1995, p. 10). This value of personal agency is incompatible with the traditional psychotherapeutic approach of teaching and coaching presumed skill deficits with adolescents.

Considerable research has been conducted on psychoeducational skill-building approaches to helping adolescents. Mann and Borduin's (1991) decade review of the 1980s' research on adolescence concluded that it has been consistently shown that social skills training improves interpersonal behaviors in role-play situations with adolescents referred for emotional and behavioral problems. Few studies have assessed adolescents' social skills in more natural settings (Mann and Borduin, 1991). In addition to concerns over the generalizability of these "predetermined programs" for adolescents, I mainly concern myself with the assumption that the resources for adolescents have to be interjected into their lives from "expert" therapists. Milton Erickson was opposed to teaching people things in psychotherapy because he viewed clients as having the resources necessary to deal with their presenting problems (O'Hanlon, 1987).

At a minimum, making therapists' work accountable to the people they work with requires the constant solicitation of clients' experience of therapy and an acknowledgment of the extent to which therapists depend on feedback for guidance (White, 1991). Even though the therapist's expertise and responsibility is in creating space for dialogue (context for change), the therapist does not know ahead of time which context will be most helpful to an adolescent and his or her family without relying rather heavily on their input.

Holding parents, adolescents, and therapists accountable necessitates assuming a tentative stance so that the therapist does not seem to be taking a moralistic position. By tentative stance I am referring to the use of tentative language, both/and thinking (opposite of dichotomous, either/or thinking), and the position of not knowing. Examples of tentative language include the use of verbs and qualifiers that keep the possibility of other alternatives open. Tentative language, both/and thinking, and the not-knowing stance are all essential elements in the cocreation of the context for ongoing dialogue. To do so enhances linguistic mobility and moves the interview toward collaborative conversation rather than toward confrontation, competition, polarization, and immobility (Anderson and Goolishian, 1988).

Therapist accountability is changing with the field's move away from "private professional knowledge," whereby therapists would often work separately with the adolescents and their families, and the process of positive results would often have a mystical quality. Now, therapists are accountable to showcase the process rather than emphasizing just therapeutic outcomes so as to enhance the personal agency of adolescents and their families in future difficulties.

EVALUATING OUR PREFERRED MODELS
OF PSYCHOTHERAPY FOR PERSONAL AGENCY
AND COGNITIVE DEVELOPMENT

The primary focus of this section is to evaluate two contemporary family therapy approaches—solution-focused therapy and narrative therapy—in terms of the enhancement of personal agency and cognitive development. The reader is encouraged to examine how his or her preferred models of psychotherapy empower adolescents and fit their developmental needs.

At first glance, the relationship between cognitive development and contemporary family therapy approaches is similar to the relationship between literacy and libraries. In both cases, the former is a requirement for the latter. If you experienced difficulty drawing the connection between the two sets of terms, imagine how arduous it must be for an adolescent still in concrete operations cognitively, to try and make sense of solution-focused therapy's miracle question. This becomes an exercise in futility.

Solution-Focused Therapy

Solution-focused therapy's main premise is that no problem is static in nature because inevitably there are times when the problem is less severe, and the client overlooks the significance of that when he or she handles the problem better. Of all the contemporary family therapy approaches, solution-focused therapy fits best with adolescents who are primarily in concrete operations (see Chapter 1).

The main reason that solution-focused therapy is a good fit for those in concrete operations is the use of an operational definition of the problem. This form of brief therapy distinguished itself from some of the more long-term forms of therapy by its insistence on presenting problems that are observable, measurable, and concrete, and its tendency to shy away from abstract, vague problem definitions or goals such as "communication," "self-esteem," or "happiness." This greatly helps an adolescent in concrete operations because the problem is now within the reach of his ears, eyes, and other senses.

Noticing differences empowers clients by helping them access their own resources for change, and the intervention can be used with young children, adolescents, and adults alike (Nelson, 1998). "Noticing what is different" is an innocuous intervention designed to identify exceptions or variations to the problem pattern which then become essential in later therapeutic conversations. Because the operational definition of the problem has been made clear, half of the work of noticing what is different is already done for the "concrete thinker."

Berg and Miller's (1982) development of scaling questions in solution-focused therapy nicely anchors a difficult conversation to a scale of numbers, which leaves the operational definition of each number up to the client, and allows for many increments of progress to be described. For example, I had been experiencing some difficulty with a twelve-year-old male, Thomas, who was rather vague in how his depression was different from the previous week. I asked Thomas, "On a scale of one to ten, where one is the worst depression you remember—stay in your room all the time, have trouble concentrating, feel sad, want to sleep—and ten is the old Thomas is back—feel like doing stuff with friends, joke around more, eat with the family, and concentrate more—where would you place yourself?" His response of six allowed me to ask Thomas what he was doing that got him to think he was at about six, and what would tell him he had moved up the scale.

In situations where no exceptions to the problem can be identified to expand upon, it may be problematic to a "concrete-thinking" adolescent to use the "suppose change happened" type of questions, because these questions require the person to extend the view beyond his or her senses to possibilities that are abstract, nonreal, and an impossibility. The advantage that adolescents (in formal operations) enjoy over children when it comes to thinking about possibilities is that adolescents are able to move easily between the specific and the abstract, to generate alternative possibilities and explanations systematically, and observe with what they believe is possible (Steinberg, 1999).

Stacey and Lopston (1995) suggest that it may be helpful to think of therapy with adolescents engaged in concrete operations in terms of "ears and eyes thinking." They suggest that therapy is a primarily verbal activity that tends to make it difficult for those in concrete operations to participate in meaningful ways. Ears thinking is the traditional dependence in therapy on verbal methods of expressing and participating. Eyes thinking takes advantage of children's abilities to visualize their experience, and becomes their aid for later ears thinking (Stacey and Lopston, 1995). In therapy with adolescents of all developmental levels, it is imperative that verbal expression is not held out to be the only acceptable form of communication, as many adolescents are gifted in the fine art mediums of drawing, music, poetry, and painting. Through the sharing of other mediums of expression, adolescents are invited to more fully participate and benefit from therapy.

Lee (1997) studied treatment outcomes for solution-focused therapy and concluded that since no significant difference was found between children and family variables and goal attainment, solution-focused brief family therapy could work equally effectively with boys and girls of different age groups, who live in diverse family constellations, and have parents from different socioeconomic strata. Lee's (1997) sample size was approximately forty cases, and she sorted the cases by age groups: seven to eleven years (coincides with concrete operations stage), twelve to thirteen (beginning of formal operations), and fourteen to sixteen (formal operations). One would think that if solution-focused therapy was generally problematic to those in "concrete operations," the percentage of goal attainment in the youngest age group would be quite low, higher in the middle age group, and highest in the oldest group. As Lee (1997) discovered, the percentage of goal attainment was very stable, around 60 percent for all three groups. "Being 'supported/validated' was the most frequently mentioned helpful element. Rigid adherence to techniques can be perceived as the therapist being inflexible, rigid, too positive, artificial, and/or insensitive—all negatively related to goal attainment" (Lee, 1997, p. 14).

How a therapist deals with becoming stuck has a major bearing on whether the client will feel supported/validated. I believe that White's (1991) suggestion to solicit the client's experience of therapy is pertinent here because it makes the process of being stuck "public" and implies that the client's input in therapy is crucial. This client feedback guards against being seduced into a "knowing position" and letting the therapist's frustration "drive the process" of therapy to the client's detriment. The likelihood of getting stuck is greater when the divergence of verbal and cognitive abilities between the therapist and clients is large.

Narrative Therapy

The two main components of narrative therapy are the deconstruction of the dominant story and the process of reconstruction of a preferred, more liberating narrative (Nicholson, 1995). Narrative therapy concerns itself with dominant stories that suffocate all other possible stories that inform clients' lives. Therapists attempt to separate negative stories from the identity of the individual by using an externalization practice that serves to weaken the grasp of the oppressive narrative, and highlight other more complementary aspects of the adolescent's life.

> We find that if we have not connected with our experience of our client's experience, as Michael White defined empathy (White and Epston, 1990), we are in danger of imposing a technique without regard to its context. This can be humiliating and harmful to clients. So we spend a good bit of time paraphrasing, restating, and reflecting content and feeling before we ask clients to help us name story titles. (Hill and Scanlon, 1998, p. 76)

Hill and Scanlon (1998) preferred titles that had an ambiguous quality so that meaning could be coconstructed rather than locked in. I do find externalizing the problem to be a fairly safe way to explore its effects without implying that the adolescent is sick or bad. There is a gradual shift from the definition of the specific acts as evil to a definition of the individual as evil, so that all of his acts come to be looked upon with suspicion (Tannenbaum, 1938). One adolescent commented to me when I externalized his anger problem, "It is not a thing, you know, it is me getting angry." I shared my concern that he would be thought of badly primarily due to this anger problem, and that I was sure there was more to him than that. He agreed that the anger problem interfered in his life because it influenced the perception of others. He reported that he needed to face his reputation as a way to practice controlling his temper. This experience suggested that one should strike a balance between empowering individuals (concern for the effects of labels) and the need to hold the adolescents accountable for their actions. This is not to imply that the externalization of problematic behavior means absolving adolescents from accountability for their actions. Conversely, this externalization practice may make it easier to accept responsibility.

One of the primary goals of deconstruction of the dominant story is the search for unique outcomes. An event is unique in the sense that it could not have been predicted from the dominant story (Nicholson, 1995). For an adolescent who carries the reputation of someone often in trouble with the law, "delinquent" becomes the master status, and the aspects of this person helping grandparents around the house each weekend, being artistic, and working well with children become overlooked and insignificant. Narrative therapy is compatible with the issues of identity formation of adolescents (Chapter 3). Identity is more than occupationally defined; it embodies a person's central values, definition of relationship with others, conceptualization of connection with his or her community, and view of the relationship between self and the spiritual or transcendent (Grotevant, 1998).

I previously thought of "identity" as an individual-oriented term, though I have shifted my thinking to view identity as a social construction. Because identity formation is dependent on relationship with others, the domain of social cognition is relevant to our discussion. The growth of social thinking—generally referred to as social cognition—during adolescence is directly related to the young person's improving ability to think abstractly (Steinberg, 1999). Social cognition is rather essential in the narrative therapy approach because if an adolescent's social thinking is less developed, it is highly probable that he will not be preoccupied with much beyond his own nose. One of the major overtones of narrative therapy is the social thinking about larger societal issues, such as the hierarchical relationship of dominant groups to marginal groups based on gender, age, ethnicity, social class, culture, and sexual orientation. This level of thinking provides a much fuller consideration of one's identity in the larger context, though the prerequisite is abstract thinking and highly developed social cognition, which may be beyond some adolescents.

One sign that adolescents are capable of abstract thought is the ability to think in multiple dimensions. Being able to understand that people's personalities are not one-sided, or that social situations can have different interpretations depending on one's point of view, permits the adolescent (formal operations) to have far more sophisticated—and far more complicated—relationships with other people (Steinberg, 1999). I tend to welcome adolescents challenging their parents' view because this is usually a sign to me that the adolescents are at a point in their development where the realization of other ways of being has dawned on them. An adolescent does not accept other people's points of view unquestioningly, but instead evaluates them against other theoretically possible beliefs (Steinberg, 1999).

Grotevant and Cooper (1985) found that adolescents higher in exploration for alternatives for their future (identity exploration) demonstrated higher frequencies of self-assertion and disagreements when interacting with their parents than did adolescents rated lower in exploration. One mother of an adolescent client of mine commented, "Everything is an argument with her; she would bicker that the sky was not blue." I think it is commonplace to unfairly define adolescents as more argumentative when, in actuality, adolescents do not argue for the sake of arguing. Rather, they suddenly realize they have opinions on issues that they were previously content to defer to their parents about. It is important for therapists to consider how much of their philosophy is dependent on abstract thinking and to tailor conversations to the client's cognitive level; otherwise, frustration is likely to set in on both sides.

For adolescents to appreciate the political agenda of narrative therapy and its implication for their therapy and life, the youth must be in formal operations of cognitive development. This is clearly seen in the adolescent's increased facility and interest in thinking about interpersonal relationships, politics, philosophy, religion, and morality—topics that involve such abstract concepts as friendship, faith, democracy, fairness, and honesty (Steinberg, 1999). Narrative therapy hinges on the client's desire for equality and a democratic voice in relation to others. Why else would anyone care about an identity or dominant story pushing them around? Because of adolescents' wish to fit in socially, narrative therapy seems like a nice fit for those in formal operations.

White and Epston (1990) have done extensive work on the therapeutic use of documents in narrative therapy to solidify therapy gains and to begin forging alternative identities for clients. When persons are established as consultants to themselves, to others, and to the therapist, they experience themselves as more of an authority on their own lives, their problems, and the solutions to these problems (White and Epston, 1990). The use of documents has the potential of being a very powerful motivator for clients because it serves as a concrete reminder of previous progress during times of doubt. The tangibility of the documents makes them a suitable fit with adolescents in concrete operations. If the adolescents are invited to cowrite the letters or documents, their potential is enhanced because the adolescents are able to add their own style, language, meaning, and development level to increase its personal significance. This is one example of an aspect of narrative therapy that could be utilized in conjunction with solution-focused therapy with adolescents in concrete operations.

SUMMARY

Adolescents are often peripheral players in the therapeutic interaction of psychotherapy with families. The intent of this chapter is to invite therapists to consider how their favored philosophies of therapy highlight the personal agency of both adolescents and their families, while being mindful of concerns of mutual accountability and cognitive development. Only by a healthy irreverence for the ideas, values, and professional knowledge that inform one's work can one encourage adolescents and their families to refuse to settle for unsatisfying aspects of their lives.

Conclusion

Adolescent development systematically influences families, presenting problems, and therapy process. It is the therapists' responsibility to carefully assess common aspects of adolescent development to ensure that they are responding appropriately to their clients. By this point, therapists should be sensitive to the following aspects of adolescent development: cognitive development, emotional development, identity development, and self-esteem. Therapists should also be sensitive to the influence of attachment, parenting relationships, and peer relationships as well as adolescent risk taking (e.g., sexual behavior, alcohol and substance abuse, suicide). Although each of these topics is presented in separate chapters, adolescents are clearly influenced by each factor simultaneously. For example, many of the case examples were discussed in multiple chapters.

CONCLUDING EXAMPLE

Aspects of family therapy with Lynn and Mindy were discussed in Chapters 4 and 8. During the first session, Mindy seemed self-conscious about the one-way mirror and video cameras. She threatened to leave and insisted that therapy would be a waste of time. If I had adopted a structural approach to therapy, I might have asked Lynn to take command of the situation and assign her the task of ensuring that Mindy attend all of our sessions. Aware of the influence of egocentrism on self-consciousness, I decided against this heavy-handed approach and instead invited Mindy to be skeptical.

I suspected that Mindy was also primarily in concrete operations, so I suggested that her contributions would be important. "I really need your perspective, Mindy. If you don't come, how will I know what your side of the story is? If I don't know your side of the story, your mom and I might come up with ideas that you won't find helpful and may even make things worse in your family; so I hope you make the decision to continue attending our sessions, at least until I have a better idea about how your family operates." I tried to provide tangible, concrete reasons to attend therapy that would be important to her.

Mindy decided to participate and seemed to be an eager participant for the first couple of months. Suddenly, she declared one week that she no longer needed to attend sessions. Lynn started to strong-arm Mindy, but I decided to ask about her change of heart.

"It's your decision, of course. Therapy isn't going to be much help if you don't want to be here. I don't want to waste your time. I will miss you, though. Could you tell me why you've suddenly decided to stop coming?"

Lynn interjected with a question. "Is it because your friend was teasing you about therapy?" Lynn explained her question. "I heard one of her friends tell her that she must be crazy if she's in therapy."

"No, that's not it," Mindy insisted.

"Well, it's your decision, Mindy. I appreciate your contributions and I will miss you, but this is your decision to make." At this point in our therapy, thinking about Byng-Hall's therapeutic tasks, I hoped that we had created a secure therapy context and that I had become an attachment figure for Mindy. I wanted to support Mindy, particularly if one of her friends was teasing her about therapy. I did not intend for this to be a paradoxical intervention. I sincerely wanted, as Robert Marrs emphasizes in Chapter 11, to convey to Mindy that I would miss her and permit her to make her own decision. I did not press her for an answer in session and told her that I would respect her decision. At the conclusion of our session, I asked Mindy if I could give her a hug in case she decided not to return. Mindy did accompany the family the next week, but she still seemed a little wary.

In Chapter 5, the influence of attachment on family dynamics was discussed. Considerable time was spent in our sessions addressing individuation issues. Lynn, who you may recall was a single mother, had recently agreed to let Mindy assume responsibility for babysitting her siblings in the afternoon. Mindy initiated this process because she indicated that she was tired of spending time at her aunt's house. She also wanted to earn some extra money for accepting this responsibility.

I was concerned that this might interfere with Mindy's ability to spend time with friends and participate in extracurricular activities. I shared an observation and asked a general question to prompt discussion. "I know that Mindy wants to baby-sit her sisters, but I'm concerned that she won't be able to also enjoy spending time with her friends and doing things at school. How can you set this up so that she gets some time just to be a teenager?" Mindy and her mother decided that Mindy would only be responsible for her sisters three days a week so that she could still attend basketball games at school and other activities.

During the middle of our work together, Mindy and Lynn experienced a time of intense conflict. It culminated when Mindy left the house one night at midnight to attend an end-of-the-year party at a friend's house. Lynn discovered that Mindy had left the house and became frantic. She called other parents and finally discovered that Mindy was at the party. Lynn arranged to have her sister stay with the remaining children so that she could find Mindy.

I was surprised at Lynn's response to this incident. For the first time since I had interacted with the family, Lynn resorted to name-calling and personal attacks on Mindy. It surprised me when she called Mindy a "drunken slut." Mindy called her mother a "bitch." The emotional intensity was high.

"This seems to have really stirred you two up. What's going on for each of you emotionally?"

Lynn answered first. "I can't believe that she would do this. I can't believe that she would sneak out of the house at midnight, go to a party, and get drunk. What in the hell were you doing, Mindy?"

I was surprised by the intensity of the anger, so I asked about it. "This seems to have triggered something. I don't know what, but it seems to have triggered something, Lynn. Any ideas?" Her answer continued to have a sharp tone. "I spent ten years married to an abusive drunk and I'm not going to go through that again. I am not going to let her destroy this family with that kind of behavior. If she wants to get drunk, she'll have to go live with her father."

I scheduled an individual session with Lynn because I wanted to find out more about her relationship with her ex-husband, but I did not want to put her children in the position of defending their father. These individual sessions helped Lynn to differentiate from her past abusive relationship so that she could respond with appropriate consequences to Mindy.

In this case, I tried to remain sensitive to Mindy's needs and aspects of adolescent development that affected her and her family. I tried to respond to her in ways that were developmentally appropriate, normalize aspects of adolescent development to Lynn, and work to improve family communication, intimacy, and trust.

SUMMARY

Awareness of developmental themes helps us understand adolescents rather than see them as mysterious specters on the fringes of their family. Awareness of adolescent development permits us to be aware of their needs at a critical time in their lives. The themes discussed in this book are compatible with a variety of approaches to therapy, and adolescents and their families seem to respond positively to this approach.

Notes

Chapter 3

1. Gerald R. Adams, Professor of Family Relations and Human Development, Department of Family Relations and Applied Nutrition, College of Social and Applied Human Sciences, University of Guelph, Guelph, Ontario, Canada N1G 2W1. E-mail: <gadams@uoguelph.ca>.

Chapter 4

1. A copy of the scale and scoring information is available in Joel Fischer and Kevin Corcoran's (1994) excellent book *Measures for Clinical Practice* (Volume 1). It is also available on the internet at <http://www.bsos.umd.edu/socy/rosenberg.htm>. The scale may be used without obtaining explicit permission, but the Rosenberg family would like to be informed of its use. The family may be contacted by correspondence at The Morris Rosenberg Foundation, c/o Dept. of Sociology, University of Maryland, 2112 Art/Soc Building, College Park, MD 20742-1315.

2. Information about the Internal Control Index is available in a journal article published by Patricia Duttweiler in the journal *Educational and Psychological Measurement*.

Chapter 5

1. The IPPA and coding instructions are available for free from Mark T. Greenberg, Director of the Prevention Research Center at Penn State University. He can be contacted by E-mail at <mxg47@psu.edu>.

Chapter 6

1. Collins and Repinski suggest that these dimensions influence relationships with both parents and peers. Although these themes will be addressed in this chapter on parent relationships, remember that they are also relevant to the material on peer relationships in Chapter 7.

2. Epstein and colleagues (1993) use the term "masked," rather than "unclear," but "unclear" seems to be a more appropriate and parallel category.

3. Information about the McMaster Family Assessment Device is available in a journal article published by Nathan B. Epstein, Lawrence M. Baldwin, and Duane S. Bishop in the *Journal of Marital and Family Therapy*. To obtain copies of the scale, contact the Family Research Program, Butler Hospital, 345 Blackstone Boulevard, Providence, RI 92906.

4. Dr. Toni Schindler Zimmerman, Department of Human Development and Family Studies, Colorado State University, Fort Collins, Colorado 80523. Email: zimmerman@CAHS.Colostate.edu.

Chapter 7

1. These two cases were briefly mentioned in the introduction.

2. This is fairly common: adolescents who run away from home typically spend their time with a friend or at the friend's house.

3. To obtain a copy of the scale, contact Dr. Steven R. Asher, Professor of Educational Psychology, University of Illinois at Urbana-Champaign, 230B Education Building, 1310 S 6th Street, Champaign, IL 61820. His E-mail address is <s-asher@uiuc.edu>.

4. You can obtain a copy of the scale by consulting the original journal publication (Vaux et al., 1986).

Chapter 9

1. Davis integrates three models for treatment: behavioral, structural-strategic, and Bowenian family therapy.

2. In this edited volume, most of the authors discuss treatment approaches that include multiple models of therapy. In one chapter, Kaufman integrates aspects of the following approaches to family therapy: psychodynamic, structural, communications, experiential, and behavioral. A structural-strategic approach is commonly recommended by other authors in this volume.

3. Lawson and Lawson suggest that abuse of alcohol and illegal substances is caused by physiological, sociological, and psychological factors. Their integrated approach includes aspects of the following family therapies: structural, strategic, Bowenian, experiential, and behavioral.

4. Stanton and Todd adopt a structural-strategic approach that also includes aspects of family development theory.

References

Adam, K. (1985). Attempted suicide. *Psychiatry Clinical North American, 8*(2), 103-201.

Adams, G. R. (1976). Personal identity formation: A synthesis of cognitive and ego psychology. *Adolescence, 12*(46), 151-164.

Adams, G. R. and Jones, R. M. (1982). Adolescent egocentrism: Exploration into possible contributions of parent-child relations. *Journal of Youth and Adolescence, 11,* 25-31.

Adams, G. R., Jones, R. M., Schvaneveldt, J. D., and Jensen, G. O. (1982). Antecedents of affective role-taking behavior: Adolescent perceptions of parental socialization styles. *Journal of Adolescence, 5*(1), 1-7.

Ainsworth, M. D. S., Waters, E., and Wall, S. (1978). *Patterns of attachment: A psychological study of the strange situation.* Hillsdale, NJ: Lawrence Erlbaum Associates.

Alexander, J. (1988). Phases of family therapy process: A framework for clinicians and researchers. In L. C. Wynne (Ed.), *The state of the art in family therapy research: Controversies and recommendations* (pp. 175-187). New York: Family Process Press.

Allen, J. P. and Land, D. (1999). Attachment in adolescence. In J. Cassidy and P. R. Shaver (Eds.), *Handbook of attachment: Theory, research, and clinical applications* (pp. 319-335). New York: Guilford Press.

Andersen, T. (1987). The reflecting team: Dialogue and meta-dialogue in clinical work. *Family Process, 26*(4), 415-428.

Andersen, T. (1992). Relationship, language, and pre-understanding in the reflecting process. *The Australian and New Zealand Journal of Family Therapy, 13*(2), 87-91.

Anderson, H. (1995). Collaborative language systems: Toward a post-modern therapy. In R. Mikesell, D. D. Lusterman, and S. McDaniel (Eds.), *Integrating family therapy: Family psychology and systems theory* (pp. 27-44). Washington, DC: American Psychological Association.

Anderson, H. and Goolishian, H. (1988). Human as linguistic systems: Preliminary and evolving ideas about the implications for clinical theory. *Family Process, 27*(4), 371-393.

Anderson, S. C. and Mandell, D. L. (1989). The use of self-disclosure by professional social workers. *Social Casework: The Journal of Contemporary Social Work, 70*(5), 259-267.

Armsden, G. C. and Greenberg, M. T. (1987). The Inventory of Parent and Peer Attachment: Individual differences and the relationship to psychological well-being in adolescence. *Journal of Youth and Adolescence, 16*(5), 427-454.

Asher, S. R. (1990). Recent advances in the study of peer rejection. In S. R. Asher and J. D. Coie (Eds.), *Peer rejection in childhood* (pp. 3-14). New York: Cambridge University Press.

Asher, S. R. and Wheeler, V. A. (1985). Children's loneliness: A comparision of rejected and neglected peer status. *Journal of Consulting and Clinical Psychology, 53*(4), 500-505.

Barret, R. L. and Robinson, B. E. (1982). Teenage fathers: Neglected too long. *Social Work, 27*(6), 484-488.

Bateson, G. (1972). *Steps to an ecology of mind.* New York: Ballantine.

Bateson, G. (1979). *Mind and nature: A necessary unity.* New York: E.P. Dutton.

Baumrind, D. (1978). Parental disciplinary patterns and social competence in children. *Youth and Society, 9*(3), 239-276.

Beck, A., Resnick, H., and Letteri, D. (Eds.) (1974). *The prediction of suicide.* Bowie, MD: Charles Press.

Becker, W. C. (1964). Consequences of different kinds of parental discipline. In M. L. Hoffman and L. W. Hoffman (Eds.), *Review of child development research* (Vol. 1) (pp. 169-208). New York: Russell Sage Foundation.

Bell, A. and Weinberg, M. (1978). *Homosexuality.* New York: Simon and Schuster.

Berg, I. and Miller, S. (1992). *Working with the problem drinker: A solution-focused approach.* New York: Norton.

Berndt, T. J. (1996). Transitions in friendship and friends' influence. In J. A. Graber, J. Brooks-Gunn, and A. C. Petersen (Eds.), *Transitions through adolescence: Interpersonal domains and context* (pp. 57-84). Mahwah, NJ: Lawrence Erlbaum.

Beskow, J. (1979). Suicide and mental disorder in Swedish men. *Academy of Psychiatry Scandinavia (Supplement), 277,* 138.

Birtchnell, J. (1983). Psychotherapeutic considerations in the management of the suicidal patient. *American Journal of Psychotherapy, 37*(1), 24-36.

Bloom, V. (1967). An analysis of suicide at a training center. *American Journal of Psychiatry, 123*(8), 918-925.

Bowen, M. A. (1985). *Family therapy in clinical practice.* New York: Jason Aronson.

Bowling, S. M. and Werner-Wilson, R. J. (1998). How does the relationship between fathers and daughters influence the sexual behavior and attitudes of heterosexual adolescent females? Paper presented at National Council on Family Relations Annual Meeting, Milwaukee, Wisconsin.

Brainerd, C. J. (1978). *Piaget's theory of intelligence.* Englewood Cliffs, NJ: Prentice-Hall.

Brent, D. (1997). Practitioner review: The aftercare of adolescents with deliberate self-harm. *Journal of Child Psychology and Psychiatry, 38*(3), 277-286.

Brent, D., Kolko, D., Wartella, M., Boylan, M., Moritz, G., Baugher, M., and Zelenak, J. (1993). Adolescent psychiatric inpatients' risk of suicide attempt at six month follow-up. *Journal of the American Academy of Child and Adolescent Psychiatry, 32*(1), 95-105.

Brook, D. W. and Brook, J. S. (1992). Family processes associated with alcohol and drug use and abuse. In E. Kaufman and P. Kaufmann (Eds.), *Family therapy of drug and alcohol abuse* (pp. 15-33). Boston, MA: Allyn and Bacon.

Brooks, R. (1994). Humor in psychotherapy: An invaluable technique with adolescents. In E. S. Buckman (Ed.), *The handbook of humor* (pp. 53-73). Malabar, FL: Krieger Publishing Company.

Brown, B. B., Clasen, D. R., and Eicher, S. A. (1986). Perceptions of peer pressure, peer conformity dispositions, and self-reported behavior among adolescents. *Developmental Psychology, 22*(4), 521-530.

Byng-Hall, J. (1995). Creating a secure family base: Some implications of attachment theory for family therapy. *Family Process, 34*(1), 45-58.

Byng-Hall, J. (1999). Family therapy and couple therapy: Toward greater security. In J. Cassidy and P. R. Shaver (Eds.), *Handbook of attachment: Theory, research, and clinical applications* (pp. 625-645). New York: Guilford Press.

Byrne, D. E. (1977). A pregnant pause in the sexual revolution. *Psychology Today, 11*(2), 67-68.

Califano, J. A. and Booth, A. (1998). *1998 CASA national survey of teens, teachers and principals.* New York: The National Center on Addiction and Substance Abuse at Columbia University.

Cannon-Bonaventure, K. and Kahn, J. (1979). Interviews with adolescent parents. *Children Today, 8*(1), 17-19.

Cassidy, J. (1999). The nature of the child's ties. In J. Cassidy and P. R. Shaver (Eds.), *Handbook of attachment: Theory, research, and clinical applications* (pp. 3-20). New York: Guilford Press.

Centers for Disease Control (1985). Suicide-United States, 1970-1980. *Morbidity and Mortality Weekly Report, 34*(24) (June 21), 353-361.

Cheung, P. C. and Lau, S. (1985). Self-esteem: Its relationship to the family and school social environments among Chinese adolescents. *Youth and Society, 16*(4), 438-456.

Cobb, C. L. H. (1996). Adolescent-parent attachments and family problem-solving. *Family Process, 35*(1), 57-82.

Cohen-Sandler, R., Berman, A., and King, R. (1982). Life-stress and symptomatology: Determinants of suicidal behavior in children. *Journal of American Academy of Child Psychiatry, 21*(2), 178-186.

Coie, J. D. (1990). Toward a theory of peer rejection. In S. R. Asher and J. D. Coie (Eds.), *Peer rejection in childhood* (pp. 365-401). New York: Cambridge University Press.

Collins, W. A. and Repinski, D. J. (1994). Relationships during adolescence: Continuity and change in interpersonal perspective. In R. Montemayor, G. R. Adams, and T. P. Gullotta (Eds.), *Personal relationships during adolescence* (pp. 7-36). Thousand Oaks, CA: Sage.

Combrinck-Graham, L. (1989). Accountability in family therapy involving children. *Journal of Psychotherapy and the Family, 6* (3/4), 9-27.

Conger, J. J. (1971). A world they never knew: The family and social change. *Daedalus, 100*(4), 1105-1138.

Cooley, C. H. (1956). *Human nature and social order.* Glencoe, IL: Free Press. (Original work published in 1902.)

Coopersmith, S. (1967). *The antecedents of self-esteem.* San Francisco, CA: W. H. Freeman.

Cowan, P. A., Powell, D., and Cowan, C. P. (1998). Parenting interventions: A family systems perspective. In W. Damon (Series Ed.) and I. E. Sigel and K. A. Renninger (Vol. Eds.), *Handbook of child psychology, Vol. 4: Child psychology in practice,* Fifth edition (pp. 5-72). New York: John Wiley and Sons, Inc.

Damon, W. (1983). *Social and personality development: Infancy through adolescence.* New York: Norton.

Damon, W. and Hart, D. (1988). *Self-understanding in childhood and adolescence.* New York: Cambridge University Press.

Davis, D. I. (1987). *Alcoholism treatment: An integrative family and individual approach.* New York: Gardner Press.

De Lissovoy, V. (1973). High school marriages: A longitudinal study. *Journal of Marriage and the Family, 35*(2), 245-255.

de Shazer, S., Berg, I. K., Lipchik, E., Nunnally, E., Molnar, A., Gingerich, W., and Weiner-Davis, M. (1986). Brief therapy: Focused solution development. *Family Process, 25*(2), 207-222.

de Shazer, S. and Molnar, A. (1984). Four useful interventions in brief family therapy. *Journal of Marital and Family Therapy, 10*(3), 297-304.

Doherty, W. J. and Colangelo, N. (1984). The family FIRO model: A modest proposal for organizing family treatment. *Journal of Marital and Family Therapy, 10*(1), 19-29.

Duttweiler, P. (1984). The Internal Control Index: A newly developed measure of locus of control. *Educational and Psychological Measurement, 44*(2), 209-221.

East, P. L., Felice, M. A., and Morgan, M. C. (1993). Sisters' and girlfriends' sexual childbearing behavior: Effects on early adolescent girls' sexual outcomes. *Journal of Marriage and the Family, 55*(4), 953-963.

Elkind, D. (1967). Egocentrism in adolescence. *Child Development, 38*(4), 1025-1034.

Epstein, N. B., Baldwin, L. M., and Bishop, D. S. (1983). The McMaster Family Assessment Device. *Journal of Marital and Family Therapy, 9*(2), 171-180.

Epstein, N. B., Bishop, D., Ryan, C., Miller, I., and Keitner, G. (1993). The McMaster Model of Family Functioning: View of healthy family functioning. In F. Walsh (Ed.), *Normal family processes,* Second edition (pp. 138-160). New York: Guilford Press.

Erikson, E. H. (1968). *Identity: Youth and crisis.* New York: W. W. Norton.

Eskilson, A., Wiley, G., Muehlbauer, G., and Doder, L. (1986). Parental pressure, self-esteem and adolescent reported deviance: Bending the twig too far. *Adolescence, 21*(83), 501-515.

Fisch, R., Weakland, J., and Segal, L. (1982). *The tactics of change: Doing therapy briefly.* San Francisco, CA: Jossey-Bass.

Fischer, J. and Corcoran, K. (1994). *Measures for clinical practice* (Vols. 1 and 2), Second edition. New York: Free Press.

Framo, J. L. (1982). *Explorations in marital and family therapy.* New York: Springer Publishing.

Freeman, J. and Combs, G. (1996). *Narrative therapy: Social construction of preferred realities.* New York: Norton.

Friedman, E. H. (1991). Bowen theory and therapy. In A. S. Gurman and D. P. Kniskern (Eds.), *Handbook of family therapy, Vol. II* (pp. 134-170). New York: Brunner/Mazel.

Furgusson, D. and Lynskey, M. (1995). Suicide attempts and suicide ideation in a birth cohort of 16-year-old New Zealanders. *Journal of the American Academy of Child and Adolescent Psychiatry, 34*(10), 1308-1317.

Furstenberg, F. F. Jr. (1976). The social consequences of teenage pregnancy. *Family Planning Perspective, 8*(4), 148-164.

Furstenberg, F. F. Jr., Levine, J. A., and Brooks-Gunn, J. (1990). The children of teenage mothers: Patterns of early childbearing in two generations. *Family Planning Perspectives, 22*(2), 54-61.

George, C., Kaplan, N., and Main, M. (1984). *Adult attachment interview protocol.* Unpublished manuscript, University of California at Berkley.

Gerber, G., Gross, L., Morgan, M., and Signorielli, N. (1986). Living with television: The dynamics of the cultivation hypothesis. In J. Bryant and D. Zillmann (Eds.), *Perspectives on media effects* (pp. 17-40). Hillsdale, NJ: Erlbaum.

Goldenstein, E. G. (1994). Self disclosure in treatment: What therapists do and don't talk about. *Clinical Social Work Journal, 22*(4), 417-433.

Goldenstein, E. G. (1997). To tell or not to tell: The disclosure of events in the therapist's life to the patient. *Clinical Social Work Journal, 25*(1), 41-58.

Goldney, R. and Bottrill, A. (1980). Attitudes to patients who attempt suicide. *Medical Journal of Australia, 2*(13), 717-720.

Greenberg, B. S., Brown, J. D., and Buerkel-Rothfuss, N. L. (1993). *Media, sex, and the adolescent.* Cresskill, NJ: Hampton Press.

Greenberg, L. S. and Johnson, S. M. (1988). *Emotionally focused therapy for couples.* New York: Guilford.

Greenberg, L. S. and Safran, J. D. (1987). *Emotion in psychotherapy.* New York: Guilford Press.

Grotevant, H. D. (1998). Adolescent development in family contexts. In W. Damon (Series Ed.) and N. Eisenberg (Vol. Ed.), *Handbook of child psychology, Vol. 3: Social, emotional, and personality development,* Fifth edition (pp. 1097-1149). New York: John Wiley and Sons, Inc.

Grotevant, H. and Cooper, C. (1985). Patterns of interaction in family relationships and the development of identity exploration. *Child Development, 56*(2), 415-428.

Haley, J. (1980). *Leaving Home.* New York: McGraw-Hill.

Hare-Mustin, R. (1987). The problem of gender in family therapy theory. *Family Process, 26*(1), 15-33.

Harter, S. (1990). Self and identity development. In S. S. Feldman and G. R. Elliot (Eds.), *At the threshold: The developing adolescent* (pp. 352-387). Cambridge, MA: Harvard University Press.

Harter, S. (1993). Causes and consequences of low self-esteem in children and adolescents. In R. F. Baumeister (Ed.), *Self-esteem: The puzzle of low self-regard* (pp. 87-116). New York: Plenum Press.

Harter, S. (1998). The development of self-representations. In W. Damon (Series Ed.) and N. Eisenberg (Vol. Ed.), *Handbook of child psychology, Vol. 3: Social, emotional, and personality development,* Fifth edition (pp. 553-617). New York: John Wiley and Sons, Inc.

Harter, S. and Marold, D. B. (1993). The directionality of the link between self-esteem and affect: Beyond causal modeling. In D. Ciccheti and S. L. Toth (Eds.), *Rochester symposium on developmental psychopathology: Disorder and dysfunctions of the self,* Vol. 5 (pp. 333-370). Rochester, NY: University of Rochester Press.

Harter, S., Marold, D. B., Whitesell, N. R., and Cobbs, G. (1996). A model of the effects of perceived parent and peer support on adolescent false self behavior. *Child Development, 67*(2), 360-374.

Hatfield, E. and Rapson, R. (1990). Emotions: A trinity. In E. A. Blechman (Ed.), *Emotions and the family: For better or for worse* (pp. 11-33). Hillsdale, NJ: Lawrence Erlbaum.

Hawton, K. and Catalan, J. (1987). *Attempted suicide: A practical guide to its nature and management.* New York: Oxford University Press.

Hawton, K., Osborn, M., O'Grady, J., and Cole, D. (1982). Classification of adolescents who take overdoses. *British Journal of Psychiatry, 140*(2), 124-131.

Hill, A. and Scanlon, C. (1998). Opening space and the two-story technique. *Journal of Family Psychotherapy, 9*(1), 75-79.

Hill, M. (1970). Suicidal behavior in adolescents and its relationship to the lack of parental empathy. *Dissertation Abstracts International, 31*(a-A), 472.

Hoff, L. (1984). *People in crisis: Understanding and helping,* Second edition. Menlo Park, CA: Addison-Wesley Publishing Co.

Hogan, D. P. and Kitagawa, E. M. (1985). The impact of social status, family structure, and neighborhood on the fertility of black adolescents. *American Journal of Sociology, 90*(4), 825-855.

Huston, A. C., Donnerstein, E., Fairchild, H., Fesbach, N. D., Katz, P. A., Murray, J. P., Rubenstein, E. A., Wilcox, B. L., and Zuckerman, D. (1992). *Big world, small screen: The role of television in American society.* Lincoln, NE: University of Nebraska Press.

Igoe, J. (1991). Empowerment of children and youth for consumer self-care. *American Journal of Health Promotion, 6*(1), 55-65.

Inhelder, B. and Piaget, J. (1958). *The growth of logical thinking from childhood to adolescence.* New York: Basic Books.

Jay, K. and Young, A. (1979). *The gay report: Lesbians and gay men speak out about sexual experience and lifestyles.* New York: Summit.

Jenson, L. C., DeGaston, J. F., and Weed, S. E. (1994). Societal and parental influences on adolescent sexual behavior. *Psychological Reports, 75*(2), 928-930.

Joanning, H. (1992). Integrating cybernetics and constructivism into structural-strategic family therapy for drug abusers. In E. Kaufman and P. Kaufmann (Eds.), *Family therapy of drug and alcohol abuse,* Second edition (pp. 94-104). Boston, MA: Allyn and Bacon.

Johnson, B., Shulman, S., and Collins, W. (1991). Systemic patterns of parenting as reported by adolescents: Developmental differences and implications for psychosocial outcomes. *Journal of Adolescent Research, 6*(2), 235-252.

Jorgensen, S. R. (1981). Sex education and the reduction of adolescent pregnancies: Prospects for the 1980s. *Journal of Early Adolescence, 1*(1), 38-52.

Kaminer, Y., Feinstein, C., and Barret, R. (1987). Suicidal behavior in mentally retarded adolescents: An overlooked problem. *Child Psychiatry and Human Development, 18*(2), 90-94.

Kapur, S., Mieczkowski, T., and Mann, J. (1992). Antidepressant medications and the relative risk of suicide attempt and suicide. *Journal of the American Medical Association, 268*(24), 3441-3445.

Kaufman, E. and Kaufmann, P. (Eds.) (1992). *Family therapy of drug and alcohol abuse,* Second edition. New York: Allyn and Bacon.

Keith, D. and Whitaker, C. A. (1987). Failure: Our bold companion. In M. Baldwin and V. Satir (Eds.), *The use of self in therapy* (pp. 8-23). Binghamton, NY: The Haworth Press.

Kerfoot, M., Dyer, E., Harrington, V., Woodham, A., and Harrington, R. (1996). Correlates and short term course of self-poisoning in adolescents. *British Journal of Psychiatry, 168*(1), 38-44.

Kirchler, E., Palmonari, A., and Pombeni, M. L. (1993). Developmental tasks and adolescents' relationships with their peers and their family. In S. Jackson and H. Rodriguez-Tomé (Eds.), *Adolescence and its social worlds* (pp. 145-167). Hillsdale, NJ: Lawrence Erlbaum.

Kobak, R. R. and Sceery, A. (1988). Attachment in late adolescence: Working models, affect regulation, and representations of self and others. *Child Development, 59*(1), 135-146.

Kohut, H. (1971). *The analysis of the self.* New York: International University Press.

Kohut, H. (1977). *The restoration of the self.* New York: International University Press.

Kosky, R., Silburn, S., and Zubrick, S. (1990). Are children and adolescents who have suicidal thoughts different from those who attempt suicide? *Journal of Nervous and Mental Disease, 178*(1), 38-43.

Landau-Stanton, J. and Stanton, M. D. (1991). Treating suicidal adolescents and their families. In M. Mirkin and S. Koman (Eds.), *Handbook of adolescents and family therapy* (pp. 273-328). New York: Gardner Press.

Lawson, A. and Lawson, G. (1998). *Alcoholism and the family: A guide to treatment and prevention,* Second edition. Gaithersburg, MD: Aspen Publishers.

Lee, M. (1997). A study of solution-focused brief family therapy: Outcomes and issues. *The American Journal of Family Therapy, 25*(1), 3-17.

Litman, R., Farbarow, N., Wold, C., and Brown, T. (1974). Prediction models of suicidal behaviors. In A. Beck, H. Resnick, and D. Letteri (Eds.), *The prediction of suicide*. Bowie, MD: Charles Press.

Maccoby, E. and Martin, J. (1983). Socialization in the context of the family: Parent-child interaction. In E. M. Hetherington (Ed.), *Handbook of child psychology: Socialization, personality, and social development*, Vol. 4. New York: Wiley.

Madigan, S. (1997). Re-considering memory: Re-membering lost identities back toward re-membered selves. In C. Smith and D. Nylund (Eds.), *Narrative therapies with children and adolescents* (pp. 338-355). New York: Guilford.

Main, M., Kaplan, N., and Cassidy, J. (1985). Security in infancy, childhood, and adulthood: A move to the level of representation. *Monographs of the Society for Research in Child Development, 50*(1-2), 66-104.

Main, M. and Solomon, J. (1990). Procedures for identifying infants as disorganized/disoriented during the Ainsworth strange situation. In M. T. Greenberg, D. Cicchetti, and E. M. Cummings (Eds.), *Attachment in the preschool years: Theory, research and intervention* (pp. 121-160). Chicago: University of Chicago Press.

Mann, B. and Borduin, C. (1991). A critical review of psychotherapy outcome studies with adolescents: 1978-1988. *Adolescence, 26*(103), 505-541.

Marcia, J. E. (1966). Development and validation of ego identity status. *Journal of Personality and Social Psychology, 3*(5), 119-133.

Marcia, J. E. (1980). Identity in adolescence. In J. Adelson (Ed.), *Handbook of adolescent psychology* (pp. 159-187). New York: Wiley.

Margolin, N. and Teicher, J. (1968). Thirteen male suicide attempts: Dynamic considerations. *Journal of the American Academy of Child Psychiatry, 7*(2), 296-315.

Marten, R., Cleninger, R., Guze, S., and Clayton, T. (1985). Mortality on a follow-up of five hundred psychiatric outpatients. *Archives of General Psychiatry, 42*(1), 58-66.

Merrell, K. W. and Gimpel, G. A. (1998). *Social skills of children and adolescents: Conceptualization, assessment, treatment*. Mahwah, NJ: Lawrence Erlbaum.

Miller, B. C., Christensen, C. R., and Olson, T. D. (1987). Adolescent self-esteem in relation to sexual attitudes and behavior. *Youth and Society, 19*(1), 93-111.

Miller, B. C., McCoy, J. K., and Olson, T. D. (1986). Dating age and stage as correlates of adolescent sexual attitudes and behavior. *Journal of Early Adolescent Research, 1*(3), 361-371.

Miller, B. C., McCoy, J. K., Olson, T. D., and Wallace, C. M. (1986). Parental discipline and control attempts in relation to adolescent sexual attitudes and behavior. *Journal of Marriage and the Family, 48*(3), 503-512.

Minuchin, S. (1974). *Families and family therapy*. Cambridge, MA: Harvard University Press.

Minuchin, S. and Fishman, H. C. (1981). *Family therapy techniques.* Cambridge, MA: Harvard University Press.

Mishne, J. (1996). Therapeutic challenges in clinical work with adolescents. *Clinical Social Work Journal, 24*(2), 137-152.

Morgan M., Jones, E., and Owen, J. (1993). Secondary prevention of non-fatal self-harm: The green card study. *British Journal of Psychiatry, 163*(1), 111-112.

Motto, J. (1978). Recognition, evaluation, and management of persons at risk for suicide. *Personnel and Guidance Journal, 56*(9), 537-543.

Mounts, N. and Steinberg, L. (1995). An ecological analysis of peer influence on adolescent grade point average and drug use. *Developmental Psychology, 31*(6), 915-922.

Murry, V. M. (1992). Incidence of first pregnancy among black adolescent females over three decades. *Youth and Society, 23*(4), 478-506.

Mussen, P. (1979). *The psychological development of the child,* Third edition. Englewood Cliffs, NJ: Prentice-Hall.

Napier, A. Y. and Whitaker, C. A. (1978). *The family crucible.* New York: Harper and Row.

National Center on Addiction and Substance Abuse at Columbia University. (1999a). *CASA survey: Many dads AWOL in the battle against teen substance abuse* [press release]. New York: Author.

National Center on Addiction and Substance Abuse at Columbia University. (1999b). *Back to school 1999—National survey of American attitudes on substance abuse V: Teens and their parents.* New York: Author.

Nelson, V. (1998). Notice the difference. *Journal of Psychotherapy and the Family, 9*(1), 81-84.

Nicholson, S. (1995). The narrative dance—A practice map for White's therapy. *Australian and New Zealand Journal of Family Therapy, 16*(1), 23-28.

Noller, P. (1994). Relationships with parents in adolescence: Process and outcome. In R. Montemayor, G. R. Adams, and T. P. Gullotta (Eds.), *Personal relationships during adolescence* (pp. 37-77). Thousand Oaks, CA: Sage.

O'Hanlon, W. (1987). *Taproots: Underlying principles of Milton Erickson's therapy and hypnosis.* New York: Norton.

O'Hanlon, W. H. and Weiner-Davis, M. (1989). *In search of solutions: A new direction in psychotherapy.* New York: Norton.

Paikoff, R. L. and Brooks-Gunn, J. (1991). Do parent-child relationships change during puberty? *Psychological Bulletin, 110*(1), 47-66.

Pantell, R., Stewart, T., Dias, J., Wells, P., and Ross, A. (1982). Physician communication with children and parents. *Pediatrics, 3*(70), 396-402.

Patel, A. (1975). Attitudes towards self-poisoning. *British Medical Journal, 2*(5968), 426-494.

Peck, M. (1985). Crisis intervention treatment with chronically and acutely suicidal adolescents. In M. Peck, N. Farbarow, and R. Litman (Eds.), *Youth Suicide.* New York: Springer.

Pfeffer, C., Hurt, S., Kakuma, T., Peskin, J., Siefker, C., and Nagabhairava, S. (1994). Suicidal children grow up: Suicidal episodes and effects of treatment during follow-up. *Journal of the American Academy of Child and Adolescent Psychiatry, 33*(2), 225-230.

Pfeffer, C., Klerman, G., Hurt, S., Lesser, M., Peskin, J., and Siefker, C. (1991). Suicidal children grow up: Demographic and clinical risk factors for adolescent suicide attempts. *Journal of the American Academy of Child and Adolescent Psychiatry, 30*(4), 609-616.

Pipher, M. (1994). *Reviving Ophelia: Saving the selves of adolescent girls.* New York: Ballantine Books.

Plutchik, R. and Plutchik, A. (1990). Communication and coping in families. In E. A. Blechman (Ed.), *Emotions and the family: For better or for worse* (pp. 35-51). Hillsdale, NJ: Lawrence Erlbaum.

Postrado, L. T. and Nicholson, H. J. (1992). Effectiveness in delaying the initiation of sexual intercourse in girls aged 12-14: Two components of the Girls Incorporated Preventing Adolescent Pregnancy Program, *Youth and Society, 23*(3), 356-379.

Proctor, J. (1959). Countertransference phenomena in the treatment of severe character disorders in children and adolescents. In Judith Mishne (Ed.), Therapeutic challenges in clinical work with adolescents. *Clinical Social Work Journal, 24*(2), 137-152.

Ramon, S. and Breyter, C. (1978). Attitudes towards self-poisoning among British and Israeli doctors and nurses in a general hospital. *Israeli Annals of Psychiatry, 16*(3), 206-218.

Ramsey, R., Tanney, B., Tierney, R., and Lang, W. (1993). *A suicide intervention training program: Trainer's handbook.* Calgary, Alberta: Living Works Education, Inc.

Reid, J., Macchetto, P., and Foster, S. (1999). *No safe haven: Children of substance-abusing parents.* New York: The National Center on Addiction and Substance Abuse at Columbia University.

Reinhertz, H., Giacona, R., Silverman, A., Friedman, A., Pakiz, B., Frost, A., and Cohen, E. (1995). Early psychosocial risks for adolescent suicidal ideation and attempts. *Journal of American Academy of Child and Adolescent Psychiatry, 34*(5), 599-611.

Resnick, M. D., Bearman, P. S., Blum, R. W., Bauman, K. E., Harris, K. M., Jones, J., Tabor, J., Beuhring, T., Sieving, R. E., Shew, M., Ireland, M., Bearinger, L. H., and Udry, J. R. (1997). Protecting adolescents from harm: Findings from the national longitudinal study on adolescent health. *Journal of the American Medical Association, 278*(10), 823-832.

Richman. J. (1979). The family therapy of attempted suicide. *Family Process, 18*(2), 131-142.

Riley, T., Adams, G. R., and Nielsen, E. (1984). Adolescent egocentrism: The association among imaginary audience behavior, cognitive development, and parental support and rejection. *Journal of Youth and Adolescence, 13*(5), 401-417.

Robins, E., Murphy, G., Wilkinson, R., Gassner, S., and Kayes, J. (1959). Some clinical observations in the prevention of suicide based on a study of 134 successful suicides. *American Journal of Public Health, 49,* 888-889.

Rodgers, J. L., Rowe, D. C., and Harris, D. F. (1992). Sibling differences in adolescent sexual behavior: Inferring process models from family composition patterns. *Journal of Marriage and the Family, 54*(1), 142-152.

Rosenberg, M. (1963). Parental interest and children's self-conception. *Sociometry, 26*(1), 35-49.

Rosenberg, M. (1979). *Conceiving the self.* New York: Basic Books.

Rosenberg, M. (1985). Self-concept and psychological well-being in adolescence. In R. L. Leahy (Ed.), *The development of the self* (pp. 205-246). New York: Academic Press.

Saarni, C. and Crowley, M. (1990). The development of emotion regulation: Effects on emotional state and expression. In E. A. Blechman (Ed.), *Emotions and the family: For better or for worse* (pp. 53-73). Hillsdale, NJ: Lawrence Erlbaum.

Saghir, M. and Robins, E. (1973). *Male and female homosexuality: A comprehensive investigation.* Baltimore, MD: Williams and Wilkins.

Sanders, G. F. and Mullis, R. L. (1988). Family influences on sexual attitudes and knowledge as reported by college students. *Adolescence, 23*(92), 837-846.

Scheck, D. C., Emerick, R., and El-Assal, M. M. (1973). Adolescents' perceptions of parent-child relations and the development of internal-external control orientation. *Journal of Marriage and the Family, 35*(4), 643-645.

Seiffge-Krenke, I. and Shulman, S. (1993). Stress, coping and relationships in adolescence. In S. Jackson and H. Rodriguez-Tomé (Eds.), *Adolescence and its social worlds* (pp. 169-196). Hillsdale, NJ: Lawrence Erlbaum.

Selzer, M. L. (1971). The Michigan Alcoholism Screening Test: The quest for a new diagnostic instrument. *American Journal of Psychiatry, 127*(12), 89-94.

Selzer, M. L., Vinokur, A., and van Rooijen, L. (1975). A self-administered Short Michigan Alcoholism Screening Test. *Journal of Studies on Alcohol, 36*(1), 117-126.

Shneidman, E. (1984). Aphorisms of suicide and some implications for psychotherapy. *American Journal of Psychotherapy, 38*(3), 319-328.

Simpson, M. (1975). Self-injury: The phenomenology of self-mutilation in a general hospital setting. *Canadian Psychiatric Association Journal, 20*(6), 429-434.

Slater, J. and Depue, R. (1981). The contribution of environmental events and social supports to suicide attempts in primary depressive disorder. *Journal of Abnormal Psychology, 90*(4), 275-285.

Smetana, J. (1995). Context, conflict, and constraint in adolescent-parent authority relationships. In M. Killen and D. Hart (Eds.), *Morality in everyday life: Developmental perspectives.* Cambridge, England: Cambridge University Press.

Stacey, K. and Lopston, C. (1995). Children should be seen and not heard? Questioning the unquestioned. *Journal of Systemic Therapies, 14*(4), 16-31.

Stanton, M. D. and Todd, T. C. (Eds.) (1982). *The family therapy of drug abuse and addiction.* New York: Guilford Press.

Stanton, M. D., Todd, T. C., Heard, D. B., Kirschner, S., Klieman, J. I., Mowatt, D. T., Riley, P., Scott, S. M., and Van Deusen, J. M. (1982). A conceptual model. In M. D. Stanton and T. C. Todd (Eds.), *The family therapy of drug abuse and addiction* (pp. 7-30). New York: Guilford.

Steinberg, L. (1999). *Adolescence*, Fifth edition. Boston: McGraw-Hill.

Stevenson, J. M. (1988). Suicide. In J. A. Talbott, R. E. Hales, and S. C. Yudofsky (Eds.), *The American Psychiatric Press textbook of psychiatry* (pp. 1021-1035). Washington, DC: The American Psychiatric Press.

Stolorow, R.D., Brandchaft, B., and Atwood, G.E. (1994). *The intersubjective perspective*. Northvale, NJ: Jason Aronsen.

Strasburger, V. C. (1995). *Adolescents and the media: Medical and psychological impact*. Thousand Oaks, CA: Sage Publications.

Tannenbaum, F. (1938). The dramatization of evil. In F. Tannenbaum (Ed.), *Crime and the Community* (pp. 19-20). New York: Columbia University Press.

Taylor, E. and Stansfeld, S. (1984). Children who poison themselves: I: A clinical comparison with psychiatric controls. *British Journal of Psychiatry, 145,* 127-132.

Thornton, A. (1990). The courtship process and adolescent sexuality. *Journal of Family Issues, 11*(3), 239-273.

Vaux, A., Phillips, J., Holly, L., Thompson, B., Williams, D., and Stewart, D. (1986). The Social Support Appraisals (SSA) Scale: Studies of reliability and validity. *American Journal of Community Psychology, 14*(2), 195-219.

Vaz-Leal, F. (1989). Psychotherapeutic management of suicide attempts in children and early adolescents: Working with parents. *Psychotherapy and Psychosomatics, 52*(1-3), 125-132.

Wassenaar, D. (1987). Brief strategic family therapy and the management of adolescent Indian parasuicide patients in the general hospital setting. *South African Journal of Psychology, 17*(3), 93-99.

Wells, L. E. and Marwell, G. (1976). *Self-esteem*. Beverly Hills, CA: Sage Publications.

Werner-Wilson, R. J. (1998a). Are virgins at-risk for contracting HIV/AIDS? *Journal of HIV/AIDS Prevention and Education for Adolescents and Children,* 2(3-4), 63-71.

Werner-Wilson, R. J. (1998b). Gender differences in adolescent sexual attitudes: The influence of individual and family factors. *Adolescence, 33*(131), 519-531.

Werner-Wilson, R. J. and Coughlin-Smith, S. (1997). How can mothers and fathers become involved in the sexuality education of adolescents in a diverse and changing world? Paper presented at National Council on Family Relations Annual Meeting. Arlington, Virginia, November.

Werner-Wilson, R. J. and Murphy, M. J. (1999). Instrumental versus expressive functions. In C. A. Smith (Ed.), *The encyclopedia of parenting theory and research* (pp. 234-235). Westport, CT: Greenwood Press.

Werner-Wilson, R. J. and Vosburg, J. (1998). How do contextual factors and gender differences influence college students' safer sex practices? *Journal of HIV/AIDS Prevention and Education for Adolescents and Children,* 2(2), 33-49.

Westley, W. A. and Epstein, N. B. (1969). *The silent majority*. San Francisco: Jossey-Bass.

Wheat, W. (1960). Motivational aspects of suicide in patients during and after psychiatric treatment. *Southern Medical Journal, 53*(3), 273-278.

Whitaker, C. A. and Keith, D. V. (1991). Symbolic-experiential family therapy. In A. S. Gurman and D. P. Kniskern (Eds.), *Handbook of family therapy, Vol. I* (pp. 187-225). New York: Brunner/Mazel.

Whitbeck, L. B., Conger, R. D., and Kao, M. Y. (1993). The influence of parental support, depressed affect, and peers on the sexual behaviors of adolescent girls. *Journal of Family Issues, 14*(2), 261-278.

White, M. (1991). Deconstruction and therapy. *Dulwich Centre Newsletter, 3,* 21-40.

White, M. (1995). *Re-authoring lives: Interviews and essays*. Adelaide, South Australia: Dulwich Centre Publications.

White, M. (1997). *Narratives of therapists' lives*. Adelaide, South Australia: Dulwich Centre Publications.

White, M. and Epston, D. (1990). *Narrative means to a therapeutic end*. New York: Norton.

Wills, T. A. (1990). Social support and the family. In E. A. Blechman (Ed.), *Emotions and the family: For better or for worse* (pp. 75-98). Hillsdale, NJ: Lawrence Erlbaum.

Wills, T. A., Blechman, E. A., and McNamara, G. (1996). Family support, coping, and competence. In E. M. Hetherington and E. A. Blechman (Eds.), *Stress, coping, and resiliency in children and families* (pp. 107-133). Mahwah, NJ: Lawrence Erlbaum.

Wilson, R. J. (1990). Are the times a'changin'? A content analysis of *Rolling Stone* magazine, 1968 and 1988. Southern Sociological Society Annual Meeting. Louisville, Kentucky, March.

Wright, D. W., Peterson, L. R., and Barnes, H. L. (1990). The relation of parental employment and contextual variables with sexual permissiveness and gender role attitudes of rural early adolescents. *Journal of Early Adolescence, 10*(3), 382-398.

Zee, H. (1972). Blind spots in recognizing serious intentions. *Bulletin of the Menninger Clinic, 36*(5), 551-555.

Zillmann, D. (1982). Television and arousal. In D. Pearl, L. Bouthilet, and J. Lazar (Eds.), *Television behavior: Ten years of scientific progress and implications for the eighties*. Vol. 2: Technical reviews (pp. 53-67). Washington, DC: U.S. Government Printing Office.

Zimmerman, T. S., Jacobsen, R. B., MacIntyre, M., and Watson, C. (1996). Solution focused parenting groups: An empirical study. *Journal of Systemic Therapies, 15*(4), 12-25.

Index

Printed in the United States
by Baker & Taylor Publisher Services